Thyroid Disease in Pregnancy - A Guide to Clinical Management

Haritha Sagili
Jayaprakash Sahoo
Swaramya Chandrasekaran
Editors

Thyroid Disease in Pregnancy - A Guide to Clinical Management

Springer

Editors
Haritha Sagili
Dept. of Obstetrics and Gynaecology
JIPMER
Puducherry, India

Jayaprakash Sahoo
Dept. of Endocrinology
JIPMER
Puducherry, India

Swaramya Chandrasekaran
Dept. of Obstetrics and Gynaecology
Sri Venkateswaraa Medical College
Hospital and Research Centre
Puducherry, India

ISBN 978-981-99-5422-3 ISBN 978-981-99-5423-0 (eBook)
https://doi.org/10.1007/978-981-99-5423-0

This Springer imprint is published by the registered company Springer Nature Singapore Pte Ltd.
The registered company address is: 152 Beach Road, #21-01/04 Gateway East, Singapore 189721, Singapore

Paper in this product is recyclable.

Preface

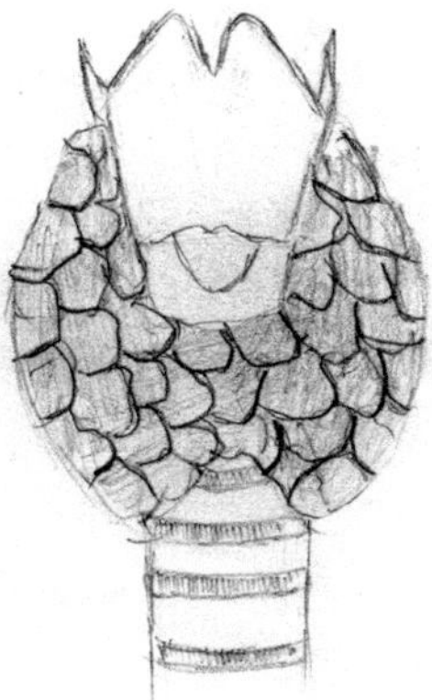

Thyroid disorders affect more women than men, with one in every eight women being likely to develop thyroid dysfunction in her lifetime. This statistic is of most relevance to practising Obstetricians and Physicians, as we wouldn't be far off the target while suspecting the most ubiquitous and overtreated condition encountered is probably thyroid centric. At various stages in our career, each of us would likely have second-guessed ourselves on starting thyroid medications for infertility or in pregnancy and peripartum. This inspired a liaison between our team Obstetricians and Endocrinologists, which birthed this clinical guide on management of thyroid disorders. We decided to write a book keeping in mind the needs of doctors, focussed on being objective and succinct. A wide range of disorders in pregnancy including hyperthyroidism and hypothyroidism, iodine supplementation, pre-conceptional management have been included. Alongside, less frequently encountered conditions like auto-immune thyroiditis and thyroid malignancies have been discussed. Practical concerns incorporating both specialties have been addressed with simple algorithms incorporating the latest evidence available. We hope this book brings as much joy and understanding of the subject, better patient management, as it did to us during hours of meticulous research.

Puducherry, India

Haritha Sagili
Jayaprakash Sahoo
Swaramya Chandrasekaran

Contents

Iodine Deficiency and Supplementation in Pregnancy and Postpartum

1

Niya Narayanan, Varun Suryadevara,
and Dukhabandhu Naik

1.1 Introduction

Iodine is a necessary micronutrient for thyroid hormone (TH) synthesis, and having enough TH is vital for proper growth and development. Also, iodine has a direct thyroid-independent role in neural development and plasticity in the postnatal period [1]. Iodine deficiency (ID) can have a variety of poor outcomes on growth and development, particularly in pregnant women and their children. Iodine deficiency disorders (IDD) is the aggregate term for these outcomes [2]. Despite considerable global measures for prevention and management, ID is still a major public health concern. ID during pregnancy is the most significant preventable cause of low intelligence quotient (IQ) in the offspring [2].

1.2 Iodine Physiology in Pregnancy

The iodine content of a healthy adult body varies between 15 and 20 mg, with 70–80% exclusively localized in the thyroid gland [3]. To maintain TH synthesis, an adult thyroid gland traps around 60–95 mcg of iodine per day in iodine-sufficient areas [3]. The thyroid gland has developed an intricate method for concentrating iodine from the circulation to meet the demand for optimal hormone production. The sodium/iodide symporter transports iodide into the thyroid at 20–50 times higher concentration gradient than plasma. Thyroxine (T4) and tri-iodothyronine (T3) are made up of 65% and 59% iodine, respectively [3].

N. Narayanan
Department of Endocrinology, Baby Memorial hospital, Calicut, India

V. Suryadevara · D. Naik (✉)
Department of Endocrinology, Jawaharlal Institute of Post Graduate Medical Education and Research (JIPMER), Puducherry, India

H. Sagili et al. (eds.), *Thyroid Disease in Pregnancy - A Guide to Clinical Management*, https://doi.org/10.1007/978-981-99-5423-0_1

The thyroid physiology changes dramatically during pregnancy. The factors which result in an increased need for TH and consequently iodine during pregnancy, have been summarized in Fig. 1.1.

This increased TH production needs a compensatory increase in iodine availability. Women in iodine-rich areas often start pregnancy with approximately 10–20 mg iodine stored in the thyroid gland, and the higher demands of pregnancy can be satisfied if adequate iodine intake is maintained [4]. Inadequate iodine intake can cause a spectrum of IDD in women from iodine-deficient regions in whom there are insufficient intrathyroidal iodine storage. Maternal iodine remains the only supply of iodine for the breast-fed newborn after delivery. The mammary gland concentrates and secretes iodine into breast milk to provide approximately 100 mcg/day of iodine for the newborn infant [5]. Table 1.1 shows World Health Organization (WHO) recommendations for daily iodine intake in women.

iodine intake by age group.

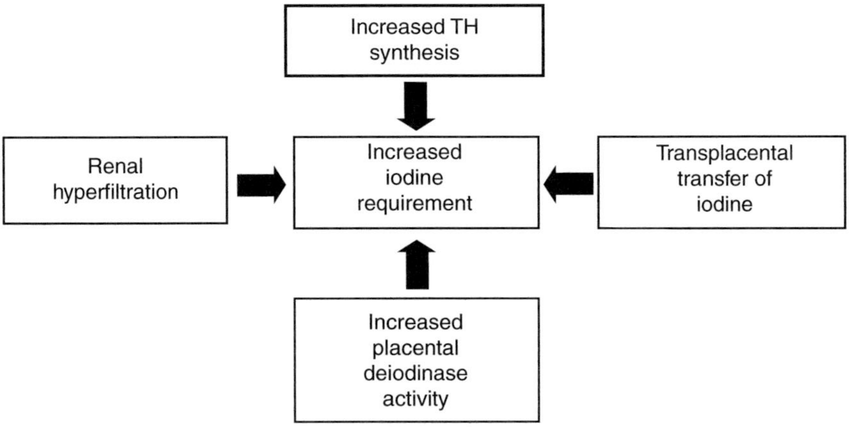

Fig. 1.1 Mechanism of increased dietary iodine requirements in pregnancy

Table 1.1 Recommendations for iodine intake in women

Population group	Daily dose of iodine intake (mcg/day)
Women of reproductive age (15–49 years)	150
Pregnant women	250
Lactating women	250

Table 1.2 Epidemiologic criteria for assessing iodine nutrition based on median urine iodine concentration

Median urinary Iodine (mcg/L)	Iodine status
Pregnant women	
<20	Severe ID
20–49	Moderate ID
50–150	Mild ID
<150	Insufficient
150–249	Adequate
250–499	Above requirements
≥500	Excessive
Lactating women	
<100	Insufficient
≥100	Adequate

ID—iodine deficiency

1.3 Definition of ID during Pregnancy and Lactation

Iodine nutrition status of the community can be measured by various approaches; median urine iodine concentration (UIC), goiter rate, serum TSH, TH, and serum thyroglobulin (TG). Because more than 90% of ingested iodine is excreted by the kidney, UIC is a sensitive predictor of recent iodine ingestion (days). Goiter prevalence is a long-term iodine nutrition (months to years) measure, whereas TG indicates an intermediate response (weeks to months) [4]. WHO recommends median UIC as the recommended test for assessing iodine intake status in populations [6]. UIC cutoffs for defining and classifying severity are presented in Table 1.2.

As studies assessing iodine levels in pregnant women are scarce, the median UIC of school-age children was used for comparison. The criterion for antenatal iodine nutrition status was modified in 2007 as recommended by WHO Technical Consultation's consensus/committee. The population median UIC cut-off of 150 μg/L was utilized to define ID in pregnancy using this revised criterion [6]. Given the greater iodine demand in pregnancy, this cut-off is higher than the median UIC levels in children and non-pregnant adults. However, there are no established cut-offs to define severity of ID in pregnancy. Thus, for research purposes, the severity of ID in pregnancy is defined as similar to that of children.

1.4 Epidemiology

According to WHO's first global estimate of goiter prevalence in 1980, ID affects 20–60% of the world's population, with the majority of the burden falling on developing countries. However, ID received little attention at first since goiter was viewed as mostly a cosmetic issue at the time. This situation changed between 1970 and 1990 when the IDD spectrum was identified, and since then, IDD elimination has been a key component of many national nutrition programs. To classify national iodine status, the median UIC is employed. In 152 nations, comprising 98% of the world's population, national UIC surveys have been conducted. In 2021, a total of 118 countries have appropriate iodine nutrition, while 21 countries are still iodine deficient. There is no severe ID in any of the countries surveyed. Surprisingly, high iodine consumption has been observed in 13 countries. For 42 nations, no UIC data is available [7].

1.4.1 Current Burden of IDD in India

IDD is a public health concern across all Indian states and union territories, according to nationwide surveys undertaken since the 1950s. 337 of the 414 districts studied all over India IDD are endemic, meaning that IDDs affect more than 5% of the population [8]. The Indian population is susceptible to ID due to a lack of iodine in the subcontinent's soil and, as a result, the food derived from it. Because they consume salt with insufficient iodine, an estimated 350 million people are at risk of developing IDD. In India, IDD affects 9 million pregnant women and 8 million newborns every year [9].

1.5 Effect of Severe ID on Pregnant Women and Their Offspring

1.5.1 Maternal and Fetal Adverse Outcomes

Miscarriage, stillbirth, neonatal death, and growth retardation are all linked to severe ID during pregnancy [10]. Kemp was the first to describe a link between ID and stillbirth in 1939 [11]. In a randomized clinical trial done in New Guinea, Pharoah et al. discovered that antenatal iodine supplementation mitigated the incidence of stillbirths and infant death [12]. When compared to those with severe ID (UIC < 50 mcg/L), women with iodine sufficiency (UIC 150–249 mcg/L) had lower incidences of preeclampsia [odds ratio(OR) = 0.12; 95% confidence interval(CI) 0.01–0.87], placenta previa [OR = 0.06; 95% CI 0.01–0.69], and fetal distress [OR = 0.10; 95% CI 0.02–0.64] [13].

Pregnant women with a UIC of <50 mcg/L had a greater chance of having a small for gestational age (SGA) baby than women with mild iodine shortage [OR = 0.15; 95 percent CI 0.03–0.76] [14]. Pregnant women who were given oral iodized oil soon before or during conception had significantly increased placental and birth weights associated with lower rates of abortion (0% vs 19%), prematurity (10.8% vs. 14.3%), and stillbirth (9.0% vs. 20.4%) [15]. Torlinska et al., on the other hand, looked at 3140 singleton pregnancies from the Avon Longitudinal Study of Parents and Children (ALSPAC) and found no link between severe ID and adverse feto-maternal outcomes like preeclampsia, gestational diabetes, glycosuria, anemia, postpartum hemorrhage, SGA, preterm delivery, or large for gestational age [16]. Maternal hypothyroxinemia can occur as a result of severe ID. Iodine supplementation during pregnancy has been demonstrated to lessen the risk of maternal hypothyroxinemia in studies. In areas with severe ID, increased rates of goiter and thyroid nodules have been recorded during pregnancy, and iodine supplementation has resulted in a reduction in maternal thyroid size [10].

During the first 20 weeks of pregnancy, the fetus is exclusively reliant on its mother for TH and iodine supply. T4 is converted to T3 by placental deiodinases, which then cross the placenta and plays an important role in fetal neurodevelopment. T3 modulates the transcription and translation of genes involved in axonal and dendritic cell proliferation, migration, synapse formation, and myelination by activating its receptor. As a result, sufficient TH is critical for fetal development, and severe ID is linked to significant and irreversible fetal abnormalities. Severe ID might have an impact on the anthropometric parameters, thyroid function, nutritional status, and mortality of newborns. Iodine supplementation in pregnant women residing in areas with severe ID has shown increased head circumference, reduced rates of microcephaly, and decreased goiter size in infants at birth [10].

1.5.2 Neonatal and Infant Survival Rates

Iodine supplementation reduces the prevalence of undernutrition and death in neonates, infants, and toddlers in areas with severe ID. Pharoah et al. tested the efficacy of a single intramuscular iodine injection in a placebo-controlled trial and found that the iodized oil-injected group had a lower neonatal mortality rate (13.3%) than the untreated group (18.2%) [12].

1.5.3 Neurocognitive Delay and Neurological Abnormalities in Offspring

Cretinism is the most well-known complication of severe ID, and its severity is determined by the time of onset and degree of hypothyroxinemia. Approximately 4–10% of severely iodine-deficient pregnant mothers have a child with cretinism [10]. The clinical phenotype of neurological cretinism includes cognitive delay, hearing and speech problems (varying degrees of deaf muteness), squint, poor voluntary motor activity (spastic diplegia or paresis of the lower limbs), and stance disorders (spastic gait and ataxia) [17].

Antenatal Iodine replacement in locations with severe ID in Papua New Guinea and Zaire provided the evidence linking severe ID to cretinism. Iodine supplementation with oral iodized oil reduced the prevalence of endemic cretinism at 4 years [risk ratio (RR) = 0.27; 95% CI 0.12–0.60] and 10 years [RR = 0.17; 95% CI 0.05, 0.58] in these studies [17, 18]. At 72 months, the children of iodine-treated mothers showed superior psychomotor development scores (91 ± 13 vs. 82 ± 14) [18]. Studies have shown that iodine supplementation in early pregnancy reduces the negative consequences of severe ID on the nervous system, while intervention later in the course of pregnancy could not reverse the impairment of neurological status. A meta-analysis in 2005 summarized the effects of Iodine on Chinese children's intellectual development, showing a profound intelligence deficit in children exposed to severe ID, with a loss of 12.45 IQ points. The IQ of their children could be raised by 8.7 points if adequate iodine supplementation was ensured before and during gestation [19].

1.6 Impact of Mild-Moderate Iodine Deficiency in Pregnancy

The evidence supporting the adverse effects of mild/moderate ID is not as strong as it is for severe ID. In pregnant women, mild/moderate iodine shortage increases thyroid volume and raises the risk of goiter [20]. Iodine supplements can help to prevent these side effects [21]. Mild/moderate ID is not associated with any significant alterations in thyroid function tests during pregnancy [21]. In a recent comprehensive analysis, researchers looked at the effects of maternal iodine supplementation on prenatal and postnatal growth and development, and found no significant differences in growth parameters between the iodine-supplemented and non-supplemented groups [22]. Due to inconsistent results from current observational research, the extent to which modest maternal iodine insufficiency during pregnancy affects the child's neurobehavioral development is still debated [20]. Observational studies have found that children born to a mother with mild maternal iodine insufficiency have a lower IQ or educational evaluation score [23, 24]. However, in a recent randomized, placebo-controlled trial, mildly iodine-deficient pregnant women in iodine-sufficient locations were randomly assigned (1:1) to receive 200 mcg iodine orally once a day or placebo until birth. The verbal and performance IQ scores of these women's offspring at ages 5–6 years were similar in both groups [25].

1.7 Iodine Prophylaxis during Pregnancy and Postpartum

The iodine prophylaxis strategy for pre-conceptional and pregnant women as recommended by the WHO depends on household coverage with iodized salt and the effectiveness of iodine prophylaxis programs adopted in each country or society. According to those factors, countries can be categorized into one of three types [6].

The different categories of countries and the strategies of iodine prophylaxis in pregnancy for each category are presented in Table 1.3.

According to WHO and Endocrine Society guidelines, women of reproductive age should consume 150 mcg of iodine per day on average, and this should be escalated to 250 mcg per day during pregnancy and breastfeeding [26, 27]. The American Thyroid Association's guidelines [28] recommend a similar intake of iodine during pregnancy, as well as the use of a single dose of 400 mg of oral iodized oil annually for women of childbearing age in low-resource countries where salt iodization or daily iodine supplements are not possible. Iodized oil is commonly utilized in distant and underdeveloped places where health care practitioners and iodide supplements are scarce. In general, all guidelines agree that iodine intake should be increased during pregnancy, and that daily iodine supplements should be taken before conception, during pregnancy, and during breastfeeding. However, because most women find out they are pregnant in the second half of the first trimester, they

Table 1.3 Strategies of iodine prophylaxis in pregnant and lactating women

Category of iodine status	Definition	Iodine prophylaxis recommendations: Women at reproductive age	Iodine prophylaxis recommendations: Pregnancy and lactation
Category 1	• Iodine sufficient countries • >90% of households use iodized salt • Iodine sufficiency was confirmed in surveillance studies with available data in pregnant women • Median UIC in such countries is higher than 100 mcg/L	USI	USI
Category 2	• 20–89% of households are consuming iodized salt • Salt iodization is not universal or is not regulated • Median UIC in such countries is between 20 and 100 mcg/L	Iodine supplementation: (a) Oral daily dose Of potassium iodide (150 mcg) (b) Single annual oral Dose of iodized oil containing 400 mg of iodine	Iodine supplementation[a]: (a) Oral daily dose of potassium iodide (250 mcg), or (b) Single annual oral dose of iodized oil containing 400 mg of iodine
Category 3	• Iodized salt is not available or available only to the minority population, <20% of households are using iodized salt • Median UIC is less than 20 mcg/L	Iodine supplementation: (a) Single annual oral Dose of iodized oil containing 400 mg of iodine (b) Oral daily dose of potassium (150 mcg)	Iodine supplementation[a]: (a) Single annual oral Dose of iodized oil containing 400 mg of iodine (b) Oral daily dose of potassium (250 mcg)

[a]Iodine supplement should not be given if iodized oil has been administered during the current pregnancy or up to 3 months prior to pregnancy

USI Universal salt iodization

begin taking iodine supplements later in the pregnancy. As a result, using iodine-fortified salt in the food sector is the only effective technique for eradicating iodine deficiency, particularly in pregnancy.

1.8 Salt Fortification with Iodine

The principle of IDD prevention measure is universal salt iodization (USI), or iodine fortification of salt used for human and cattle consumption, including salt used in the food industry. Iodide and iodate, usually as the potassium salt, are the two most common forms of iodine used to iodize salt. Iodate is a more stable form of iodide, thus it is better for moist tropical environments. Human salt consumption ranges from 5 to 15 grams per day, depending on culture and climate. As a result, the level of iodination in salt may vary depending on local conditions (1:25,000–1:100,000). The lowest quantity that will provide 100 mcg of Iodine per day is 30 ppm (30 mg of potassium iodate per kg of salt). Many local issues may obstruct the proper implementation of the salt fortification program. The main hurdles that have hampered successful iodination prophylaxis include inadequate iodination of salt, difficulties in obtaining potassium iodate, transportation and coordination issues with distribution initiatives, and the rural population's intake of inadequately iodinated "cattle" salt. Successful salt iodination programs need continuous surveillance of the iodized salt produced and consumed.

1.8.1 Universal Salt Iodization Status in India

In 1962, India was one of the first countries to implement salt iodization. When IDD control was included in the National Development Program in 1983, the scenario changed. The National Goiter Control Program (NGCP) was renamed as the National IDD Control Program (NIDDCP) in 1992 to emphasize the government's commitment to eradicate all forms of IDD. In India, significant progress toward universal salt iodization has been made over the last two decades [29].

Currently, the national household coverage of iodized salt (at least $\geq$5 ppm) is 92.4%. About 76.3% of households have salt with $\geq$15 ppm iodine (95%CI): 74.1–78.5%), and 16.1% of households had salt with some iodine (>5 ppm–15 ppm). Only 7.6% of the households have salt with no iodine (<5 ppm). The highest coverage of iodized salt ($\geq$15 ppm) was observed in Jammu and Kashmir (99.8%), while the lowest coverage was observed in Tamil Nadu (61.9%). In urban areas, 82.9% of the households were using iodized salt ($\geq$15 ppm) compared to only 72.2% of households in rural areas. In pregnant women, the median UIC was 173.4 mcg/L, which is well within the adequate range (i.e., between 150 and 249 mcg/L). The findings were similar across rural and urban areas, with urban areas having slightly higher median UIC (180.2 mcg/L) than rural areas (168.9 mcg/L). The median UIC among lactating women was 172.8 mcg/L [8].

1.9 Effects of Iodine Excess in Pregnancy and Postpartum

Excessive iodine consumption can have a negative impact on thyroid function in those who are vulnerable. The acute Wolff-Chaikoff effect occurs when elevated iodine levels cause transitory suppression of thyroid hormone synthesis in healthy people. Within a few days, the thyroid "escapes" from the acute Wolff-Chaikoff effect due to downregulation of the iodide transporter in thyroid cells, and normal thyroid hormone synthesis restarts. Women with underlying thyroid issues, such as thyroid autoimmunity, may not be able to overcome the acute Wolf-Chaikoff effect and may become hypothyroid when exposed to too much iodine. Thyroid function and UIC have a U-shaped relationship, according to a recent cross-sectional study from China. They hypothesized that there is a small window for adequate iodine intake during pregnancy, with UIC levels of <150 mcg/L and >250 mcg/L being linked to an increased risk of maternal hypothyroidism [30]. The ability to fully escape the acute Wolff-Chaikoff effect does not mature until 36 weeks of pregnancy, and even if maternal thyroid function is preserved, fetal hypothyroidism can develop in the presence of a high iodine load. Congenital hypothyroidism has been found to be associated with excessive maternal iodine consumption in some case reports. The use of iodine-containing antiseptics during delivery may cause transient hypothyrotropinemia or hypothyroidism in newborns. Fetuses of iodine-deficient mothers are more susceptible to increased iodine intake. Iodine-induced hyperthyroidism, on the other hand, is a failure of the acute Wolff-Chaikoff effect. This is prevalent in people with nodular goiters, and is particularly more pronounced in areas where iodine is scarce.

Key Messages

- Thyroid hormones are vital for every organ system's metabolic function as well as the fetus's neurological and somatic development.
- Iodine requirements, which are required for thyroid hormone synthesis, rise dramatically during pregnancy and lactation.
- Iodine deficiency affects 20–60% of the world's population.
- Because of the widespread adoption of USI, the prevalence of severe insufficiency has dropped considerably worldwide in recent decades.
- Worldwide, severe ID remains the major preventable cause of intellectual impairment.
- Even mild-to-moderate iodine shortage has been shown in studies to have negative impacts on maternal and neonatal outcomes.
- Based on current data, iodine supplementation is advised for pregnant, breastfeeding, and reproductive age group women in areas where mild-to-moderate iodine shortage persists.
- The iodine prophylaxis strategy for pregnant women and women planning for pregnancy depends on household coverage with iodized salt and the effectiveness of iodine prophylaxis programs adopted in each country.

- WHO and Endocrine Society guidelines recommend 150 mcg of iodine per day for women of reproductive age and 250 mcg per day during pregnancy and breastfeeding.
- Pregnant women's health providers must be aware of this critical micronutrient and encourage proper iodine intake during preconception, pregnancy, and breastfeeding.

References

1. Hetzel BS. Iodine and neuropsychological development. J Nutr. 2000;130:493S–5S.
2. Zimmermann MB, Boelaert K. Iodine deficiency and thyroid disorders. Lancet Diabetes Endocrinol. 2015;3:286–95.
3. Zimmermann MB, Jooste PL, Pandav CS. Iodine-deficiency disorders. Lancet Lond Engl. 2008;372:1251–62.
4. Werner & Ingbar's the thyroid. 11th edition. Philadelphia, PA: LWW; 2020.
5. Jameson JL, Groot LJD. Endocrinology: adult and pediatric E-book. Elsevier Health Sciences; 2015.
6. Secretariat WHO, Andersson M, Benoist B de, Delange F, Zupan J. Prevention and control of iodine deficiency in pregnant and lactating women and in children less than 2-years-old: conclusions and recommendations of the technical consultation. Public Health Nutr; 2007;10:1606–1611.
7. Iodine Global Network (IGN)–Home [Internet]. [cited 2021 Nov 16]. Available from: https://www.ign.org/cm_data
8. Directorate General Of Health Services [Internet]. [cited 2021 Nov 16]. Available from: https://dghs.gov.in/content/1348_3_NationalIodineDeficiency.aspx
9. Pandav CS, Yadav K, Srivastava R, Pandav R, Karmarkar MG. Iodine deficiency disorders (IDD) control in India. Indian J Med Res. 2013;138:418–33.
10. Toloza FJK, Motahari H, Maraka S. Consequences of severe iodine deficiency in pregnancy: evidence in humans. Front Endocrinol. 2020;11:409.
11. Kemp WN. Iodine deficiency in relation to the stillbirth problem. Can Med Assoc J. 1939;41:356–61.
12. Pharoah PO, Ellis SM, Ekins RP, Williams ES. Maternal thyroid function, iodine deficiency and fetal development. Clin Endocrinol. 1976;5:159–66.
13. Yang J, Liu Y, Liu H, Zheng H, Li X, Zhu L, et al. Associations of maternal iodine status and thyroid function with adverse pregnancy outcomes in Henan Province of China. J Trace Elem Med Biol Organ Soc Miner Trace Elem GMS. 2018;47:104–10.
14. Alvarez-Pedrerol M, Guxens M, Mendez M, Canet Y, Martorell R, Espada M, et al. Iodine levels and thyroid hormones in healthy pregnant women and birth weight of their offspring. Eur J Endocrinol. 2009;160:423–9.
15. Chaouki ML, Benmiloud M. Prevention of iodine deficiency disorders by oral administration of lipiodol during pregnancy. Eur J Endocrinol. 1994;130:547–51.
16. Torlinska B, Bath SC, Janjua A, Boelaert K, Chan S-Y. Iodine status during pregnancy in a region of mild-to-moderate iodine deficiency is not associated with adverse obstetric outcomes; results from the Avon longitudinal study of parents and children (ALSPAC). Nutrients. 2018;10:E291.
17. Thilly CH, Delange F, Lagasse R, Bourdoux P, Ramioul L, Berquist H, et al. Fetal hypothyroidism and maternal thyroid status in severe endemic goiter. J Clin Endocrinol Metab. 1978;47:354–60.

18. Cao XY, Jiang XM, Dou ZH, Rakeman MA, Zhang ML, O'Donnell K, et al. Timing of vulnerability of the brain to iodine deficiency in endemic cretinism. N Engl J Med. 1994;331:1739–44.
19. Qian M, Wang D, Watkins WE, Gebski V, Yan YQ, Li M, et al. The effects of iodine on intelligence in children: a meta-analysis of studies conducted in China. Asia Pac J Clin Nutr. 2005;14:32–42.
20. Pearce EN, Lazarus JH, Moreno-Reyes R, Zimmermann MB. Consequences of iodine deficiency and excess in pregnant women: an overview of current knowns and unknowns. Am J Clin Nutr. 2016;104(Suppl 3):918S–23S.
21. Taylor PN, Okosieme OE, Dayan CM, Lazarus JH. Therapy of endocrine disease: impact of iodine supplementation in mild-to-moderate iodine deficiency: systematic review and meta-analysis. Eur J Endocrinol. 2014;170:R1–15.
22. Farebrother J, Naude CE, Nicol L, Sang Z, Yang Z, Jooste PL, et al. Effects of iodized salt and iodine supplements on prenatal and postnatal growth: a systematic review. Adv Nutr Bethesda Md. 2018;9:219–37.
23. Velasco I, Carreira M, Santiago P, Muela JA, García-Fuentes E, Sánchez-Muñoz B, et al. Effect of iodine prophylaxis during pregnancy on neurocognitive development of children during the first two years of life. J Clin Endocrinol Metab. 2009;94:3234–41.
24. Murcia M, Rebagliato M, Iñiguez C, Lopez-Espinosa M-J, Estarlich M, Plaza B, et al. Effect of iodine supplementation during pregnancy on infant neurodevelopment at 1 year of age. Am J Epidemiol. 2011;173:804–12.
25. Gowachirapant S, Jaiswal N, Melse-Boonstra A, Galetti V, Stinca S, Mackenzie I, et al. Effect of iodine supplementation in pregnant women on child neurodevelopment: a randomised, double-blind, placebo-controlled trial. Lancet Diabetes Endocrinol. 2017;5:853–63.
26. WHO | Iodine supplementation in pregnant and lactating women [internet]. WHO. World Health Organization; [cited 2021 Nov 17]. Available from: https://www.who.int/elena/titles/guidance_summaries/iodine_pregnancy/en/
27. De Groot L, Abalovich M, Alexander EK, Amino N, Barbour L, Cobin RH, et al. Management of thyroid dysfunction during pregnancy and postpartum: an Endocrine Society clinical practice guideline. J Clin Endocrinol Metab. 2012;97:2543–65.
28. Alexander EK, Pearce EN, Brent GA, Brown RS, Chen H, Dosiou C, et al. 2017 guidelines of the American thyroid association for the diagnosis and management of thyroid disease during pregnancy and the postpartum. Thyroid Off J Am Thyroid Assoc. 2017;27:315–89.
29. Kaur G, Anand T, Bhatnagar N, Kumar A, Jha D, Grover S. Past, present, and future of iodine deficiency disorders in India: need to look outside the blinkers. J Fam Med Prim Care. 2017;6:182–90.
30. Shi X, Han C, Li C, Mao J, Wang W, Xie X, et al. Optimal and safe upper limits of iodine intake for early pregnancy in iodine-sufficient regions: a cross-sectional study of 7190 pregnant women in China. J Clin Endocrinol Metab. 2015;100:1630–8.

Preconceptional Management of Thyroid Disease

2

K. G. Rashmi and Jayaprakash Sahoo

2.1 Introduction

Thyroid disorders are common in women of childbearing age. Overt thyroid dysfunction is known to increase the risk of adverse pregnancy outcomes, such as miscarriage, stillbirth, and neuro-intellectual impairment in the offspring. These adverse events, however, can also occur in patients with subclinical hypothyroidism (SCH) and isolated hypothyroxinemia, albeit to a lesser extent. Prompt correction of thyroid dysfunction is crucial for preventing adverse effects on maternal and fetal outcomes. The thyroid hormones play a key role in intrauterine fetal growth and neuronal development. During early gestation, the fetus is completely dependent on maternal thyroxine until 14–18 weeks, when the fetus begins to secrete thyroid hormones [1]. At this early stage of fetal life, several critical developmental events occur such as proliferation and migration of neurons, and neural tube formation. Thus, it represents the most vulnerable period during which maternal thyroid dysfunction could have long-lasting repercussions [1]. In order to optimize thyroid disease outcomes in pregnancy, effective treatment before conception is imperative. This chapter highlights the pragmatic approach to preconception management of women with thyroid disease.

Authors' Contributions: KGR has drafted the book chapter. Both authors have edited and approved the final manuscript.

K. G. Rashmi · J. Sahoo (✉)
Department of Endocrinology, JIPMER, Puducherry, India

H. Sagili et al. (eds.), *Thyroid Disease in Pregnancy - A Guide to Clinical Management*, https://doi.org/10.1007/978-981-99-5423-0_2

Types of Thyroid Dysfunction

1. Hypothyroidism (subclinical and overt).
2. Isolated hypothyroxinemia.
3. Euthyroid autoimmunity.
4. Assisted reproduction technology (ART) and thyroid dysfunction.
5. Hyperthyroidism.

2.1.1 Hypothyroidism

Overt hypothyroidism is defined by low free thyroxine (FT4) levels with elevated thyroid stimulating hormone (TSH). It affects 0.3%–0.5% of the population and is ten times more prevalent in women than men [2]. In iodine-rich countries, primary hypothyroidism is mainly due to autoimmune or Hashimoto's thyroiditis, which is distinguished by the presence of thyroid-specific antibodies such as thyroid peroxidase Ab (TPOAb) and thyroglobulin Ab (TgAb) in the circulation. However, iodine deficiency continues to be the most prevalent cause of primary hypothyroidism globally. Other causes include radioiodine therapy or thyroidectomy for benign and malignant thyroid disease. Overt hypothyroidism due to any cause increases the risk of adverse pregnancy outcomes such as miscarriage (1.8–4 fold), eclampsia, anemia, preterm birth, and lower intelligent quotient (IQ) in the child by up to seven points [3]. Studies have shown that controlling overt hypothyroidism significantly improves fetal survival rates when TSH levels are kept within the target range [4, 5]. Currently, there is insufficient data to suggest universal screening of TSH levels before conception, except for women planning assisted reproduction or those with TPOAb positivity [6].

Preconception Management of Hypothyroidism

The aims of preconception management include correcting pre-existing hypothyroidism, offering preconception counselling, and increasing levothyroxine (LT4) dosage prior to conception.

- The full dose of LT4 (0.8–1.6 μg/kg/day) therapy should be started in women with recently diagnosed hypothyroidism, and they should be counselled regarding compliance to treatment and the necessity of optimizing thyroid hormone replacement prior to conception. Patients should be reassured that the use of LT4 is safe during pregnancy and that appropriate replacement will result in a satisfactory pregnancy outcome. Women treated with LT4 should have a preconception TSH target of between the lower reference limit and 2.5 mU/L, similar to the first-trimester target. Liothyronine or desiccated thyroid supplements are not recommended in the preconception period and during pregnancy as it contains lower T4/T3 (thyroxine/tri-iodothyronine) ratio compared to normal thyroid gland. Therefore, transplacental passage of maternal T4 to fetal brain may be insufficient. In addition, T3 is completely degraded in the placenta [7].

- Hypothyroid women planning for pregnancy should check their TSH levels, and LT4 dosage must be adjusted to achieve a value between the lower reference limit and 2.5 mU/L [6].
- LT4 dose titration should be done as soon as pregnancy is confirmed to reduce the chance of maternal hypothyroidism. The aim is to normalize TSH concentrations throughout the pregnancy. The dose of LT4 could be increased empirically in several ways, such as doubling of LT4 dose twice a week, which could be a 30% increase [8] or increasing the LT4 dose by 50% in patients receiving more than 100 μg daily and by 25% in those receiving less than 100 μg daily [9]. Alternatively, LT4 dose can be increased by approximately 25%–30% [6]. There is evidence that aiming for a low-normal TSH before conception guarantees a postconception TSH of 2.5 mU/L, but it needs to be confirmed whether this approach is safe in non-specialist settings [10, 11].

Summary of Preconception plan [7]

1. Monitor TSH and FT4.
2. The LT4 dose should be titrated to target TSH.
3. Postpone pregnancy until FT4 and TSH are in the target range.
4. Emphasize on treatment adherence.
5. Offer specific guidance on conception.
    - Seek medical advice if pregnancy is suspected, such as a missed period or a positive pregnancy test.
    - To check TSH and FT4.
    - LT4 dose should be increased before the blood test results are available. For example, A. Double the daily dose of LT4 twice a week, such as 100 μg Monday through Friday and 200 μg Saturday and Sunday or B. Increase the dose of LT4 by 25 μg daily if receiving ≤100 μg daily (125 μg) and by 50 μg if receiving >100 μg (150 μg).
    - Avoid taking LT4 with antenatal vitamin supplements, iron tablets, or antacids.

Case Scenario 1

A 31-year-old female, on treatment for overt hypothyroidism for 5 years, married for 2 years, currently on tab thyroxine 100 μg daily, recent serum TSH—4 mU/L, planning for pregnancy. What will be the plan of management?

Answer: Increase the LT4 dose by 25 μg daily.

2.1.2 Subclinical Hypothyroidism (SCH)

Contrary to overt hypothyroidism, it is unclear whether Subclinical Hypothyroidism (SCH) patients (elevated TSH with normal FT4 levels) should receive LT4. SCH affects 2–3% of pregnant women, although a higher rate has been reported when stringent upper TSH cut offs are used [12]. Progression rates from subclinical to overt disease are 2–5% per year and are increased in individuals with TSH >10 mU/L or positive TPOAb [2]. The adverse feto-maternal outcomes associated with overt hypothyroidism are also observed in SCH [5]. In observational studies, SCH has been linked with a higher risk of miscarriage, placental abruption, preterm delivery, and stillbirth [13–15]. Recent research from a national health program in China (n = 184,611 women) revealed that TSH >2.5 mU/L in the 6 months prior to conception was associated with a significant risk of miscarriages and preterm birth [16]. Although the risk of these adverse outcomes is generally much lower than in overt hypothyroidism, the high prevalence of SCH makes it a relevant public health problem. SCH has primarily been associated with a higher risk of adverse obstetric outcomes but there are few data to suggest an association with adverse neurobehavioral outcomes in offspring [17].

The effects of treatment of SCH during pregnancy remain unclear. Two main outcomes have been studied, namely child neurodevelopment and obstetric outcomes. Regarding child neurodevelopment, most large prospective observational studies show that hypothyroxinemia but not SCH is associated with child IQ or brain imaging outcomes. Two recent large randomized controlled trials (RCTs) have studied the effects of LT4 treatment in women with SCH during pregnancy on child IQ, but neither study found any beneficial effects [18, 19].

For women with SCH, there is no data to guide decision-making on LT4 treatment. A first step would be to verify that SCH is persistent by rechecking serum TSH and FT4 concentrations after 3 months [20]. In agreement with most international guidelines, treatment is recommended in women with TSH >10 mU/L, and treatment is considered in those with any of the risk factors for thyroid dysfunction such as [6]:

1. Current symptoms/signs of thyroid disease or past history of hyperthyroidism or hypothyroidism.
2. Presence of goiter or TPO Ab positivity.
3. History of prior thyroid surgery or radiation to head and neck.
4. Recent use of lithium, amiodarone, or administration of iodinated radiologic contrast agent.
5. Living in an iodine insufficient area.

If LT4 treatment is not started, clinical follow-up throughout gestation is warranted. All patients planning for pregnancy or who are already pregnant should undergo a clinical evaluation, and testing for serum TSH is advised if any risk factors are present [6]. It is important to remember that the definition of SCH during the preconception period should be based on the reference range for nonpregnant women rather than the ATA-recommended TSH target of 2.5 mU/L for women with established hypothyroidism. Additionally, borderline results should be re-evaluated 6–8 weeks later before making a diagnosis [7].

Case Scenario 2

A 30-year-old female, no past history of thyroid disorder, married for 3 years, routine health check revealed serum TSH—6 mU/L (Normal: 0.27–4.2) with normal T4 and T3, planning for pregnancy. What is the diagnosis and treatment option for thyroid dysfunction?

Answer: SCH. Start treatment with LT4.

2.2 Isolated Hypothyroxinemia

Isolated hypothyroxinemia refers to the biochemical finding of normal TSH concentration with low FT4 levels [21]. The etiology of this condition is unclear. The prevalence depends on the diagnostic FT4 threshold used and the iodine nutritional status of the population and ranges from 1% to 10% in iodine-sufficient countries to 20–30% in iodine-deficient areas [22]. Isolated hypothyroxinemia has been linked with adverse neuro-behavioral outcomes in the offspring, such as language delay, autism, schizophrenia, attention deficit hyperactivity disorders, a slower reaction time, suboptimal academic performance, lower cortical volume, and gray matter [16]. Pop et al. reported that infants born to women with persistent hypothyroxinemia at 12-week gestation showed an 8–10 point deficit in mental and motor function scores compared to the offspring of euthyroid mothers [23]. It is unclear whether isolated hypothyroxinemia has been associated with bad obstetric outcomes [24]; with some studies have reported this association while others have not [25].

There is currently no evidence that correcting hypothyroxinemia with LT4 has any beneficial effects on a child's neuro-intellectual function. The two RCTs that have looked at this issue so far found no evidence that mothers with gestational hypothyroxinemia benefit from LT4 on their child's IQ [18, 19, 26]. ATA 2017 guidelines recommend against routine treatment. Individual risk factors such as a history of pregnancy complications or other comorbidities as well as the potential risk for overtreatment should be taken into account during individualized clinical decision-making [6].

2.3 Euthyroid Autoimmunity

Approximately 10% of pregnant women have TPOAb positivity without any evidence of thyroid dysfunction, although prevalence rates vary depending on race and iodine intake [27]. Thyroid autoimmunity is more common in women with infertility and recurrent miscarriages [28], and about a fifth of untreated TPOAb-positive women develop overt hypothyroidism during pregnancy [29]. Results from meta-analyses show that maternal thyroid autoimmunity disease increases the overall risk of miscarriage in both spontaneous and assisted pregnancies [30–32]. Some proposed mechanisms are innate thyroid hormone deficiency, the activation of a widespread autoimmune process leading to fetal allografts rejection, and the confounding effects of TPOAb positivity in older women [33]. Additionally, dissociation between hCG and FT4 levels has been observed in TPOAb-positive women at high risk of preterm delivery, raising the possibility that TPOAb positivity may impair the thyroid's response to hCG [34]. Whether LT4 treatment can prevent fetal loss in TPOAb-positive women has not been established. Negro et al. showed that miscarriage rates were higher in untreated TPOAb-positive euthyroid pregnant women compared to TPOAb-positive women who received LT4 therapy (13.8 vs 3.5%) [29]. There is insufficient data regarding whether LT4 treatment improves fertility in nonpregnant, euthyroid, TPOAb-positive women attempting conception naturally. Thyroid function tests (TFT) should be monitored during pregnancy because of the risk of thyroid dysfunction [6].

2.4 ART and Thyroid Dysfunction

TFTs remain stable throughout a normal menstrual cycle, but controlled ovarian hyperstimulation (COH) protocols have clear effects on thyroid physiology. The rapid increase in estradiol during COH raises thyroxine-binding globulin (TBG) concentrations to the same extent as during pregnancy and increases type 3 deiodinase (D3) gene transcription [35]. Therefore, an increase in thyroid hormone production is essential to ensure adequate thyroid hormone availability. In addition, hCG administration slightly increases FT4 levels. Women treated with a fixed dosage of LT4 typically exhibit a substantial increase in TSH levels, peaking around the time of hCG stimulation, but do not exhibit the increase in FT4 levels as seen in non-treated women. TPOAb-positive women typically exhibit a substantial increase in TSH which remains high thereafter, while the FT4 levels seem to decline only slightly toward the end of the COH course [36, 37].

- TFT should be performed either before or 1–2 weeks after COH, as the results obtained during COH may be difficult to interpret [6].
- Euthyroid TPOAb positive undergoing ART: The observational studies have demonstrated that TPOAb positivity is linked with an approximately 44% higher risk of miscarriage and, consequently, also with a 35% lower relative probability of live birth [31]. Although TPOAb-positive women appear to be at higher risk of miscarriage, there is no evidence to support LT4 treatment for euthyroid TPOAb-positive women undergoing ART. This is supported by the results of a large RCT performed in China that included euthyroid TPOAb-positive women undergoing in vitro fertilization (IVF) treatment. Compared to an equally sized control group, 226 women who received LT4 (25–50 μg/day, depending on their TSH concentration) had similar rates of miscarriage (10.6 vs. 10.3%) and live births (32.3 vs. 31.7%) [38]. These results are partly replicated by the TABLET trial performed in the UK [39] in which 45% of the included euthyroid TPOAb-positive women underwent fertility treatments and no benefit of LT4 treatment could be identified. Therefore, there seems to be no indication for preconception LT4 treatment for euthyroid TPOAb-positive women, and only clinical follow-up from early pregnancy onward seems warranted.

- Overt hypothyroidism requires thyroid hormone replacement with a preconception or pre-ART target TSH of <2.5 mU/L. It is advised to counsel patients to contact their health care providers before starting ART or at the time of a positive pregnancy test to increase their LT4 dosage by roughly 30%.
- For women with SCH undergoing fertility treatments, the indications for LT4 treatment are less clear. TPOAb-positive SCH is considered to be a treatment indication. Decisions about LT4 treatment should take into account the presence of other risk factors for adverse ART or pregnancy outcomes, including a prior history of miscarriage or failed ART or age > 35 years. If LT4 therapy is elected, it should be started at a low dose (25–50 μg), with subsequent dose titration to a target serum TSH of <2.5 mU/L [20].

2.5 Hyperthyroidism

In countries with sufficient iodine, hyperthyroidism, or the overproduction of thyroid hormones, is diagnosed in 0.1–1.0% of all pregnancies [40]. Graves' disease is the primary cause of the vast majority of cases, though occasionally, it can be due to solitary and multiple autonomously functioning nodules [41]. Uncontrolled maternal hyperthyroidism is associated with maternal hypertension, miscarriages, stillbirths, intrauterine growth retardation, cardiac arrhythmias, and heart failure [42, 43]. Adverse effects are seen more commonly in association with overt hyperthyroidism but not with subclinical hyperthyroidism [44] which in most instances represents the normal physiological changes during pregnancy.

Preconception Management of Hyperthyroidism

Preconception care aims to reduce the risk of maternal hyperthyroidism and exposure to antithyroid drugs (ATDs) in the subsequent pregnancy [6, 45, 46]. All women of childbearing age who develop thyrotoxicosis should be discussed regarding ATD therapy during potential future pregnancies. Pregnancy should generally be delayed until a stable euthyroid state is reached [6, 45]. A stable euthyroid state can be defined using two sets of TFTs within the reference range, taken at least 1 month apart, with no change in therapy between tests. Contraception is strongly recommended until hyperthyroidism is controlled. Hyperthyroid women who desire future pregnancy may be offered medical treatment with ATD, ^{131}I ablative therapy, or thyroid surgery. Each therapeutic option has advantages and disadvantages for women with Graves' Disease planning for future pregnancy such as [6]:

1. Antithyroid drugs (ATDs)

   Advantages:

   a. Effective treatment for Euthyroidism within 12 months.
   b. Gradual remission of autoimmunity [decrease TSH receptor antibody (TRAb) titers].
   c. Can be easily discontinued.
   d. Good adherence and treatment is inexpensive.

Disadvantages:

a. Adverse effects of ATD (mild 5–8%, severe 0.2%).
b. Birth defects linked to methimazole (3–4%) and propylthiouracil (2–3%).
c. Relapse after ATD withdrawal is likely high (50%–70%).

2. Radioactive iodine (RAI) therapy.

Advantages:

a. Easy to administer orally.
b. Improvement in goiter size.
c. Relapse to hyperthyroidism is very rare.

Disadvantages:

a. Occasionally, repeat therapy may be needed.
b. Rising TRAb titers after RAI therapy may worsen orbitopathy or increase fetal risk.
c. Following RAI ablation, LT4 therapy may be necessary for lifelong.

3. Thyroidectomy.

Advantages:

a. Definitive therapy for Grave's disease.
b. A stable euthyroid state can easily be achieved by replacing LT4.
c. Gradual abatement of autoimmunity.
d. Disappearance of goiter.

Disadvantages:

a. Lifelong need for LT4 replacement.
b. Surgical complications occur in 2–5% of cases.
c. Takes time for healing and recovery from surgery.
d. Permanent scar on the neck.

Upon confirmation of the pregnancy, specific instructions should be given to all women by their healthcare practitioners. For women contemplating future pregnancy, radioiodine, or surgery can be an alternative to ATD therapy, as pregnancy may trigger a relapse following ATD treatment. In women with a high probability of relapse, for instance, those with high TRAb titers, large goiter, ophthalmopathy, and severe biochemical disease, definitive therapy is most appropriate [7] (Fig. 2.1).

For women on ATDs, the following discussion is recommended:

(a) If the patient has received ATD for more than 2 years and has a persistently elevated TRAb level, the likelihood of remission during pregnancy is low and ATD therapy is most likely required during pregnancy.
(b) Both ATDs are teratogenic, although the malformations associated with propylthiouracil (PTU) are less frequent and less severe. PTU is hepatotoxic and may induce liver failure requiring liver transplantation; therefore, it is recommended that PTU use be limited outside the pregnancy setting. In younger women with regular menses who are likely to conceive relatively quickly, switching from methimazole (MMI) to PTU before conception is advisable (Fig. 2.1).
(c) In carefully selected patients on ATD who are likely to be in remission (those without large goiters, with normal serum TSH on minimal amounts of ATD

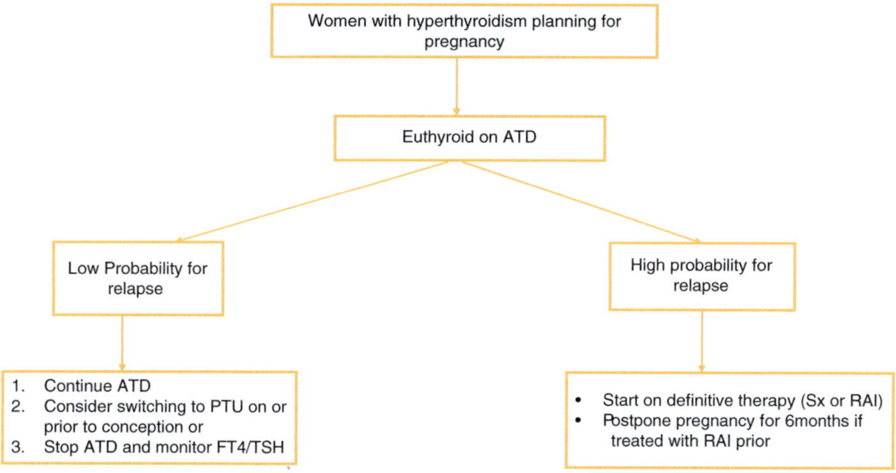

Fig. 2.1 Preconception management of Graves' disease in women planning for pregnancy. *ATD* antithyroid drugs; *LT4* levothyroxine; *PTU* propylthiouracil; *Sx* surgery; *RAI* radioactive iodine; *TRAb* TSH receptor antibody

(e.g., 2.5–5 mg of MMI a day) and without elevated TRAb titers), ATD can be continued pre-pregnancy and then stopped immediately when pregnancy is diagnosed [47] (Fig. 2.1).

Indeed, in some women who appear to be in remission with normal TRAb, the drug could be stopped before pregnancy is documented. In such patients, thyroid function should be monitored every 4–6 weeks. In patients taking MMI until conception, thyroid function and symptoms must be monitored closely, every 1–2 weeks, throughout the first trimester, and ATD restarted if necessary. The hope is that if hyperthyroidism recurs following cessation of ATD, it will do so only after the period of organogenesis when ATD therapy can be safely restarted.

(d) Close follow-up with frequent blood tests and adjustment of ATD is required throughout pregnancy as dose adjustments are often required.
(e) There is a possibility of disease exacerbation in the first trimester and exacerbation in the postpartum period [48].
(f) TRAb determination in the second trimester will be required for the prediction of potential fetal or neonatal complications.

Pregnant women who undergo ablative therapy with radioactive iodine should consider the following recommendations [6]:

- First, following ^{131}I therapy, TRAb levels rise and can remain elevated for many months. Therefore, patients with high TRAb levels or severe hyperthyroidism may benefit from considering other therapeutic options, such as surgery.
- Second, ^{131}I therapy may fail to achieve euthyroid status in a subset of young patients with Graves' disease.

- Third, if ^{131}I ablation is being planned, a pregnancy test should be done 48 h before the procedure to ensure that no unintended pregnancy has occurred.
- Fourth, pregnancy should be postponed for 6 months to ensure a stable euthyroid state following ablation, and initiating LT4 replacement therapy is considered.
- Lastly, in individuals at high risk of recurrence, a total thyroidectomy may be preferable because thyroidectomy usually, although not always, results in the disappearance of circulating TRAbs [6].

Case Scenario 3

A 32-year-old female, k/c/o Graves' disease for 3 years, married for 1 year, currently on tab carbimazole 10 mg daily, recent serum TSH–0.1 (0.5–5.5 mU/L), FT4–1.2 (0.89–1.76 ng/dL), FT3–3 (2.3–4.2 pg/mL), mild goiter, no ophthalmopathy, planning for pregnancy. What will be the plan of management?

Answer: Continue ATD and switch to PTU on conception or switch to PTU preconception or stop ATDs and monitor FT4/TSH.

Key Messages

- Thyroid disorders in women of childbearing age are becoming more common, and many of these patients need preconception counselling by Endocrinologists or general practitioners.
- With careful and practical preconception planning and treatment, the risk of thyroid dysfunction during pregnancy leading to adverse maternal and fetal outcomes can be reduced.
- More research is required to establish the best treatment strategy for women with hypothyroxinemia, euthyroid autoimmunity and subclinical hypothyroidism, as well as safe use of ATD during peri-conception.
- The debate regarding screening for thyroid disease is unlikely to be resolved without adequately powered interventional trials.

Conflict of interest Nil.

Funding Nil.

References

1. Moog NK, Entringer S, Heim C, Wadhwa PD, Kathmann N, Buss C. Influence of maternal thyroid hormones during gestation on fetal brain development. Neuroscience. 2017 Feb;7(342):68–100.
2. Vanderpump MPJ. The epidemiology of thyroid disease. Br Med Bull. 2011;99:39–51.

3. Alexander EK, Marqusee E, Lawrence J, Jarolim P, Fischer GA, Larsen PR. Timing and magnitude of increases in levothyroxine requirements during pregnancy in women with hypothyroidism. N Engl J Med. 2004 Jul 15;351(3):241–9.
4. Hallengren B, Lantz M, Andreasson B, Grennert L. Pregnant women on thyroxine substitution are often dysregulated in early pregnancy. Thyroid Off J Am Thyroid Assoc. 2009 Apr;19(4):391–4.
5. Abalovich M, Gutierrez S, Alcaraz G, Maccallini G, Garcia A, Levalle O. Overt and subclinical hypothyroidism complicating pregnancy. Thyroid Off J Am Thyroid Assoc. 2002 Jan;12(1):63–8.
6. Alexander EK, Pearce EN, Brent GA, Brown RS, Chen H, Dosiou C, et al. 2017 guidelines of the American Thyroid Association for the diagnosis and Management of Thyroid Disease during Pregnancy and the postpartum. Thyroid Off J Am Thyroid Assoc. 2017 Mar;27(3):315–89.
7. Okosieme OE, Khan I, Taylor PN. Preconception management of thyroid dysfunction. Clin Endocrinol. 2018 Sep;89(3):269–79.
8. Yassa L, Marqusee E, Fawcett R, Alexander EK. Thyroid hormone early adjustment in pregnancy (the THERAPY) trial. J Clin Endocrinol Metab. 2010 Jul;95(7):3234–41.
9. Chan S, Boelaert K. Optimal management of hypothyroidism, hypothyroxinaemia and euthyroid TPO antibody positivity preconception and in pregnancy. Clin Endocrinol. 2015 Mar;82(3):313–26.
10. Abalovich M, Alcaraz G, Kleiman-Rubinsztein J, Pavlove MM, Cornelio C, Levalle O, et al. The relationship of preconception thyrotropin levels to requirements for increasing the levothyroxine dose during pregnancy in women with primary hypothyroidism. Thyroid Off J Am Thyroid Assoc. 2010 Oct;20(10):1175–8.
11. Rotondi M, Mazziotti G, Sorvillo F, Piscopo M, Cioffi M, Amato G, et al. Effects of increased thyroxine dosage pre-conception on thyroid function during early pregnancy. Eur J Endocrinol. 2004 Dec;151(6):695–700.
12. Moreno-Reyes R, Glinoer D, Van Oyen H, Vandevijvere S. High prevalence of thyroid disorders in pregnant women in a mildly iodine-deficient country: a population-based study. J Clin Endocrinol Metab. 2013 Sep;98(9):3694–701.
13. Sheehan PM, Nankervis A, Araujo Júnior E, Da Silva CF. Maternal thyroid disease and preterm birth: systematic review and meta-analysis. J Clin Endocrinol Metab. 2015 Nov;100(11):4325–31.
14. Maraka S, Ospina NMS, O'Keeffe DT, Espinosa De Ycaza AE, Gionfriddo MR, Erwin PJ, et al. Subclinical hypothyroidism in pregnancy: a systematic review and meta-analysis. Thyroid Off J Am Thyroid Assoc. 2016 Apr;26(4):580–90.
15. Negro R, Stagnaro-Green A. Diagnosis and management of subclinical hypothyroidism in pregnancy. BMJ. 2014 Oct 6;349:g4929.
16. Chen S, Zhou X, Zhu H, Yang H, Gong F, Wang L, et al. Preconception TSH and pregnancy outcomes: a population-based cohort study in 184 611 women. Clin Endocrinol. 2017 Jun;86(6):816–24.
17. Korevaar TIM, Tiemeier H, Peeters RP. Clinical associations of maternal thyroid function with foetal brain development: epidemiological interpretation and overview of available evidence. Clin Endocrinol. 2018 Aug;89(2):129–38.
18. Lazarus JH, Bestwick JP, Channon S, Paradice R, Maina A, Rees R, et al. Antenatal thyroid screening and childhood cognitive function. N Engl J Med. 2012 Feb 9;366(6):493–501.
19. Casey BM, Thom EA, Peaceman AM, Varner MW, Sorokin Y, Hirtz DG, et al. Treatment of subclinical hypothyroidism or hypothyroxinemia in pregnancy. N Engl J Med. 2017 Mar 2;376(9):815–25.
20. Werner & Ingbar's The Thyroid: A Fundamental and Clinical Text [Internet]. [cited 2021 Nov 8]. Available from: https://www.wolterskluwer.com/en/solutions/ovid/werner%2D%2Dingbars-the-thyroid-a-fundamental-and-clinical-text-855
21. Negro R, Soldin OP, Obregon MJ, Stagnaro-Green A. Hypothyroxinemia and pregnancy. Endocr Pract Off J Am Coll Endocrinol Am Assoc Clin Endocrinol. 2011 Jun;17(3):422–9.
22. Moleti M, Trimarchi F, Vermiglio F. Doubts and concerns about isolated maternal hypothyroxinemia. J Thyroid Res. 2011;2011:463029.

23. Pop VJ, Brouwers EP, Vader HL, Vulsma T, van Baar AL, de Vijlder JJ. Maternal hypothyroxinaemia during early pregnancy and subsequent child development: a 3-year follow-up study. Clin Endocrinol. 2003 Sep;59(3):282–8.
24. Cleary-Goldman J, Malone FD, Lambert-Messerlian G, Sullivan L, Canick J, Porter TF, et al. Maternal thyroid hypofunction and pregnancy outcome. Obstet Gynecol. 2008 Jul;112(1):85–92.
25. Casey BM, Dashe JS, Spong CY, McIntire DD, Leveno KJ, Cunningham GF. Perinatal significance of isolated maternal hypothyroxinemia identified in the first half of pregnancy. Obstet Gynecol. 2007 May;109(5):1129–35.
26. Hales C, Taylor PN, Channon S, Paradice R, McEwan K, Zhang L, et al. Controlled antenatal thyroid screening II: effect of treating maternal suboptimal thyroid function on child cognition. J Clin Endocrinol Metab. 2018 Apr 1;103(4):1583–91.
27. Krassas GE, Poppe K, Glinoer D. Thyroid function and human reproductive health. Endocr Rev. 2010 Oct;31(5):702–55.
28. Poppe K, Velkeniers B, Glinoer D. The role of thyroid autoimmunity in fertility and pregnancy. Nat Clin Pract Endocrinol Metab. 2008 Jul;4(7):394–405.
29. Negro R, Formoso G, Mangieri T, Pezzarossa A, Dazzi D, Hassan H. Levothyroxine treatment in euthyroid pregnant women with autoimmune thyroid disease: effects on obstetrical complications. J Clin Endocrinol Metab. 2006 Jul;91(7):2587–91.
30. Thangaratinam S, Tan A, Knox E, Kilby MD, Franklyn J, Coomarasamy A. Association between thyroid autoantibodies and miscarriage and preterm birth: meta-analysis of evidence. BMJ. 2011 May 9;342:d2616.
31. Busnelli A, Paffoni A, Fedele L, Somigliana E. The impact of thyroid autoimmunity on IVF/ICSI outcome: a systematic review and meta-analysis. Hum Reprod Update. 2016 Nov;22(6):775–90.
32. Velkeniers B, Van Meerhaeghe A, Poppe K, Unuane D, Tournaye H, Haentjens P. Levothyroxine treatment and pregnancy outcome in women with subclinical hypothyroidism undergoing assisted reproduction technologies: systematic review and meta-analysis of RCTs. Hum Reprod Update. 2013 Jun;19(3):251–8.
33. Prummel MF, Wiersinga WM. Thyroid autoimmunity and miscarriage. Eur J Endocrinol. 2004 Jun;150(6):751–5.
34. Korevaar TIM, Steegers EAP, Pop VJ, Broeren MA, Chaker L, de Rijke YB, et al. Thyroid autoimmunity impairs the thyroidal response to human chorionic gonadotropin: two population-based prospective cohort studies. J Clin Endocrinol Metab. 2017 Jan 1;102(1):69–77.
35. Huang SA, Mulcahey MA, Crescenzi A, Chung M, Kim BW, Barnes C, et al. Transforming growth factor-beta promotes inactivation of extracellular thyroid hormones via transcriptional stimulation of type 3 iodothyronine deiodinase. Mol Endocrinol Baltim Md. 2005 Dec;19(12):3126–36.
36. Poppe K, Glinoer D, Tournaye H, Schiettecatte J, Devroey P, van Steirteghem A, et al. Impact of ovarian hyperstimulation on thyroid function in women with and without thyroid autoimmunity. J Clin Endocrinol Metab. 2004 Aug;89(8):3808–12.
37. Gracia CR, Morse CB, Chan G, Schilling S, Prewitt M, Sammel MD, et al. Thyroid function during controlled ovarian hyperstimulation as part of in vitro fertilization. Fertil Steril. 2012 Mar;97(3):585–91.
38. Wang H, Gao H, Chi H, Zeng L, Xiao W, Wang Y, et al. Effect of levothyroxine on miscarriage among women with Normal thyroid function and thyroid autoimmunity undergoing in vitro fertilization and embryo transfer: a randomized clinical trial. JAMA. 2017 Dec 12;318(22):2190–8.
39. Dhillon-Smith RK, Middleton LJ, Sunner KK, Cheed V, Baker K, Farrell-Carver S, et al. Levothyroxine in women with thyroid peroxidase antibodies before conception. N Engl J Med. 2019 Apr 4;380(14):1316–25.
40. Korevaar TIM, Medici M, Visser TJ, Peeters RP. Thyroid disease in pregnancy: new insights in diagnosis and clinical management. Nat Rev Endocrinol. 2017 Oct;13(10):610–22.

41. Carlé A, Pedersen IB, Knudsen N, Perrild H, Ovesen L, Rasmussen LB, et al. Epidemiology of subtypes of hyperthyroidism in Denmark: a population-based study. Eur J Endocrinol. 2011 May;164(5):801–9.
42. Okosieme OE, Lazarus JH. Current trends in antithyroid drug treatment of graves' disease. Expert Opin Pharmacother. 2016 Oct;17(15):2005–17.
43. Andersen SL, Olsen J, Wu CS, Laurberg P. Spontaneous abortion, stillbirth and hyperthyroidism: a Danish population-based study. Eur Thyroid J. 2014 Sep;3(3):164–72.
44. Casey BM, Dashe JS, Wells CE, McIntire DD, Leveno KJ, Cunningham FG. Subclinical hyperthyroidism and pregnancy outcomes. Obstet Gynecol. 2006 Feb;107(2 Pt 1):337–41.
45. Ross DS, Burch HB, Cooper DS, Greenlee MC, Laurberg P, Maia AL, et al. 2016 American Thyroid Association guidelines for diagnosis and Management of Hyperthyroidism and Other Causes of thyrotoxicosis. Thyroid Off J Am Thyroid Assoc. 2016 Oct;26(10):1343–421.
46. Lazarus JH. Pre-conception counselling in graves' disease. Eur Thyroid J. 2012 Apr;1(1):24–9.
47. De Leo S, Pearce EN. Autoimmune thyroid disease during pregnancy. Lancet Diabetes Endocrinol. 2018 Jul;6(7):575–86.
48. Tagami T, Hagiwara H, Kimura T, Usui T, Shimatsu A, Naruse M. The incidence of gestational hyperthyroidism and postpartum thyroiditis in treated patients with graves' disease. Thyroid Off J Am Thyroid Assoc. 2007 Aug;17(8):767–72.

3 Screening and Interpretation of Thyroid Function Tests in Pregnancy

Rajan Palui and Sadishkumar Kamalanathan

3.1 Introduction

Thyroid disease in pregnancy can affect two lives, the mother and the fetus. Thus, it is very important to diagnose thyroid diseases in early pregnancy and start the necessary treatment. Grossly, the spectrum of thyroid diseases can be grouped into hypothyroidism and thyrotoxicosis in pregnancy. There are strong evidences in favor of early diagnosis and treatment of overt disease [1]. On the other hand, there are differences in opinion relating to management of subclinical hypothyroidism, subclinical hyperthyroidism, isolated hypothyroxinemia, and euthyroid autoimmunity [2, 3]. In this chapter, we will briefly discuss the importance of early diagnosis of thyroid disease through screening tests and pros and cons of different case finding strategies. We will also discuss how the various components of thyroid function tests should be interpreted in view of altered physiology of pregnancy and a pragmatic approach to diagnose important thyroid disorders in pregnancy through these tests.

3.2 Screening for Thyroid Disorders in Pregnancy

Thyroid disorders are one of the most common endocrine disorders in pregnancy. In a recent meta-analysis, the prevalence of overt hypothyroidism, subclinical hypothyroidism, and isolated hypothyroxinemia were reported to be 0.5%, 3.5%, and 2% respectively [4]. On the other hand, the prevalence of subclinical and overt thyrotoxicosis in pregnancy were 2.5% and 0.2%, respectively [5]. It is not uncommon to

R. Palui
Department of Endocrinology, The Mission Hospital, Durgapur, India

S. Kamalanathan (✉)
Department of Endocrinology, JIPMER, Puducherry, India

H. Sagili et al. (eds.), *Thyroid Disease in Pregnancy - A Guide to Clinical Management*, https://doi.org/10.1007/978-981-99-5423-0_3

miss the diagnosis clinically, as these disorders might be completely asymptomatic or sometimes the symptoms can mimic that of normal pregnancy. Thus, it is rational to screen for thyroid disorders in early pregnancy for timely diagnosis and treatment, and also to prevent adverse maternal and fetal outcomes. The guidelines for screening thyroid disorders in pregnancy are not similar globally and differs from country to country. Two types of screening strategies are generally followed—universal screening and targeted screening among high-risk pregnant women. Universal screening is recommended by guidelines from Italy and Spain [6, 7]. On the other hand, guidelines from American Thyroid Association (ATA) [3], the American College of Obstetricians and Gynecologists [8], and countries like India [9] and Brazil [10] still recommend targeted screening strategy. High-risk pregnant women in whom routine thyroid screening is recommended as per ATA guideline is given in Table 3.1.

The advantages of universal screening will be the early identification and treatment of not only overt but also subclinical thyroid disorders. However, there are doubts about definite benefits of early treatment of subclinical disease [11] and risk of possible harm due to overtreatment [12]. The cost of universal screening will also be higher than targeted screening. On the other hand, targeted screening strategy has the risk of missing a large number of pregnancies with thyroid disorders. The "10 criteria" laid by James Wilson and Gunner Jungner, for evaluation of the need for a screening program is considered as gold standard [13]. These criteria are summarized in Table 3.2.

Taylor et al. evaluated screening of both hypothyroid and hyperthyroid disorders in pregnancy based on these above-mentioned criteria [14]. The authors found that overt thyroid disorders fulfill all the criteria for universal screening in pregnancy. However, as there is a lack of unanimous consensus for whom to treat in subclinical hypothyroidism, all except criteria number 8 (vide Table 3.2) were fulfilled for universal screening for subclinical thyroid disorders. Similarly, in another review, Stagnaro-Green et al. also reported that overt hypothyroidism fulfills all the criteria

Table 3.1 Targeted screening criteria for thyroid disorders in pregnancy (as per ATA guideline 2017) [3]

Screening with TSH is recommended in pregnancy with any of the following risk factors:
1. A history of hypothyroidism/hyperthyroidism or current symptoms/signs of thyroid dysfunction.
2. Known thyroid antibody positivity or presence of a goiter.
3. History of head or neck radiation or prior thyroid surgery.
4. Age > 30 years.
5. Type 1 diabetes or other autoimmune disorders.
6. History of pregnancy loss, preterm delivery, or infertility.
7. Multiple prior pregnancies.
8. Family history of autoimmune thyroid disease or thyroid dysfunction.
9. Morbid obesity (BMI $\geq$40 kg/m^2).
10. Use of amiodarone or lithium, or recent administration of iodinated radiologic contrast.
11. Residing in an area of known moderate to severe iodine insufficiency.

ATA American Thyroid Association; *BMI* Body Mass Index; *TSH* Thyroid stimulating hormone

Table 3.2 Wilson and Jungner criteria for evaluation of screening strategy [13]

1. Is the condition an important health problem?
2. Is there an accepted treatment?
3. Are facilities for diagnosis and treatment readily available?
4. Is there a recognizable latent or early symptomatic stage?
5. Is there a suitable test or examination?
6. Is the test acceptable to the population?
7. Is the natural history of the condition, adequately understood?
8. Is there an agreed policy on whom to treat?
9. Is the cost of case finding economically viable?
10. Case finding should be a continuing process and not a "once and for all" project.

for universal screening whereas other thyroid disorders in pregnancy meet most of the criteria [15]. Dosiou et al. evaluated the cost-effectiveness of universal screening programs with respect to targeted screening in the United States and found it to be cost-effective [16]. Even a Spanish study reported that universal screening can be cost-saving with respect to high-risk population screening [17]. Surveys among clinicians have also shown an increased trend of adopting universal screening strategies [18, 19].

As of now, ATA does not recommend universal screening due to lack of sufficient evidence (Recommendation 94) [3]. However, based on recent literature as discussed above, universal screening for thyroid disorders can improve maternal and fetal outcomes while maintaining cost-effectiveness. Majority of guidelines recommend serum thyroid stimulating hormone (TSH) as the screening test of choice, followed by measurement of thyroid hormones if indicated rather than measurement of both TSH and tetraiodothyronine (T4) together for initial assessment [3, 8].

3.3 Thyroid Function Tests in Pregnancy

Thyroid function tests (TFT) are one of the most frequently performed hormonal tests during pregnancy. Among the TFTs, TSH, and thyroid hormones—T4 and triiodothyronine (T3) are mostly required for diagnosis of different thyroid disorders in pregnancy. Apart from these, measurement of thyroid autoantibodies like anti-thyroid peroxidase (Anti-TPO) antibody, anti-thyroglobulin (Anti-Tg) antibody, and TSH receptor antibody (TRAb) are needed in limited circumstances.

Physiological changes that occur during normal pregnancy can significantly influence the measurement and interpretation of TFTs [20]. Firstly, there is a significant increase in the level of thyroid binding globulin (TBG) during pregnancy. At the end of 20 weeks of gestation, TBG rises by 2–3 times from the pre-pregnancy level. This rise is due to both increased production and decreased clearance of sialylated protein, secondary to hyperestrogenic state of pregnancy. As majority of thyroid hormones (both T3 and T4) are heavily bound with TBG, the circulating level of both total T4 and total T3 also rises by 50% at around the 16th week of gestation. Secondly, human chorionic Gonadotropin (hCG) starts rising in the first trimester of pregnancy and reaches a peak by the end of the first trimester and thereafter, it plateaus during rest of the pregnancy. There is molecular mimicry between TSH and hCG due to common "alpha unit" and thus hCG can stimulate thyrocytes by acting through the TSH receptor, leading to increased production of thyroid hormones. As a result of this, by the end of first trimester, the serum T4 level rises to the peak and consequently TSH level decreases due to the negative feedback effect on the pituitary and hypothalamus by increased circulating thyroid hormones. In the later part of pregnancy, the hCG and free T4 level gradually plateau and TSH level rises a little from its nadir.

3.3.1 Serum TSH

Measurement of serum TSH plays a pivotal role in the diagnosis of thyroid disorders. A normal TSH level can rule out almost all of the common thyroid disorders of pregnancy except a few rare disorders. However, various factors influence the true "normal" level of TSH in a pregnant woman and it varies according to the gestational age, ethnicity, method of analysis, and other factors. Normal TSH levels in pregnancy change according to the gestational age, due to the effect of physiological change of hCG levels in pregnancy as discussed above. In most of the studies, it had been reported that the TSH level reaches its nadir around 10th–11th week of gestation and thereafter slowly increases till term [21]. For this reason, ATA guideline recommends the use of trimester-specific reference range of TSH and if not available, then to reduce the lower and upper reference level by 0.4 mU/L and 0.5 mU/L, respectively [3]. Serum TSH levels can also be affected by the presence of thyroid autoimmunity. In patients with positive thyroid antibodies, TSH levels have been reported to be higher than controls [22]. Moreover, Korevaar et al. reported blunting of hCG-induced changes in thyroid hormones in patients with positive antibody status [23].

Iodine nutrition status can also affect TSH levels in pregnant women. Studies have reported higher TSH levels in pregnant mothers with severe iodine deficiency [24]. Due to various factors including prevalence of thyroid autoimmunity, normal TSH level also varies according to ethnicity. TSH levels are found to be highest among Asian and lowest among black women [25]. Normal TSH reference intervals also vary according to the methods and instruments used for the biochemical assay. Thus, considering all of these variables, ATA advocates to use population, trimester and laboratory-specific reference ranges for serum TSH. Such a normal reference range for each trimester should be developed from the TSH level measurements of at least 120 rigorously screened antibody negative, clinically euthyroid pregnant mothers with normal iodine status [26]. Presence of concurrent illness (non-thyroid illness syndrome) and concomitant use of drugs (like dopamine, glucocorticoids, and amiodarone) can also affect serum TSH levels in pregnant women. While interpreting TSH reports, clinicians should also be careful regarding the possibility of the presence of other interfering factors like presence of heterophil antibodies (can both falsely elevate or suppress TSH) and macro TSH (false elevation) molecules [27].

3.3.2 Serum Total T4/Free T4

T4 can be measured both as its bound form (total T4) as well as free T4. Both of these assays have their own advantages and limitations, specifically due to physiological alterations in pregnancy. Total T4 assay is easy to perform, widely available, and has a lesser chance of analytical interference. However, the total T4 assay results should be interpreted according to gestational age due to physiological rise of TBG in pregnancy. ATA has recommended to increase the upper reference limit of total T4 by 5% for every week from the 7th–16th week of gestation. From the 16th week of gestation onward, 1.5 times of non-pregnant reference limits can be used [3, 28]. So, for example, if total T4 is measured at 12 weeks of gestation, the reference limits should be increased by 30% (5% rise per week for 6 weeks) from nonpregnant level. Though, this formula is very pragmatic to follow in clinical practice, it may not be universally applicable [29].

Out of the total T4 in circulation, only 0.04% remains in its free form (free T4) and this free hormone is responsible for the thyroid hormone action at tissue level. As the serum concentration of free T4 remains in picomolar range, it is much more difficult to measure in comparison to total T4 which is measured in nanomolar range. Direct measurement based on the equilibrium dialysis method is still the ideal method to measure free T4, but it is not readily available except in research settings. Most commercially available assays of free T4 use indirect immunoassay methods and are highly prone to errors due to various interferences during pregnancy. Due to change in serum concentrations of binding proteins in pregnancy, the accuracy of free T4 measurement by different immunoassays has been reported to be unreliable [30]. Other factors like increase in free fatty acid levels and decreased albumin in pregnancy can also affect indirect immunoassays. Various drugs which are commonly used in pregnancy can also interfere with free T4 measurement. Drugs like heparin (by increasing circulating non-esterified fatty acids) and aspirin can spuriously increase free T4 levels by displacing it from circulating thyroid hormone binding sites [31]. Use of biotin-containing over-the-counter multivitamins can also interfere with competitive free T4 immunoassays which use biotinylated analogues [32]. Similar to TSH, the use of assay methods and trimester-specific reference ranges of free T4 have also been advocated [3]. Unfortunately, these data are not readily available for all the immunoassay techniques yet. Other methods of indirect free T4 measurements like free T4 index, T4/TBG ratios, and resin uptake methods have been tried. Free T4 can also be measured directly by more reliable liquid chromatography/mass spectrometry (LC/MS) techniques [33]. However, like equilibrium dialysis, this method is also costly and not widely available.

An individual participant data meta-analysis, which included 9036 mother–child pairs from three population-based prospective cohorts, reported maternal free T4 assessed by immunoassay as a reliable marker of maternal thyroid hormone status in early pregnancy [34]. The free T4 measured by immunoassays appeared to correlate well with the neuro-development of the child [34]. Compared to total T4, maternal free T4 has been found to be better associated with adverse maternal and fetal outcomes in pregnancy [35]. Moreover, the assay inferences associated with indirect immunoassays are usually less severe in the early period of pregnancy. In conclusion, both total and free T4 can be used as markers of maternal thyroid function during pregnancy. In the early part of pregnancy, free T4 correlates better with maternal and fetal outcomes, while in the latter half of pregnancy, total T4 with pregnancy-adjusted reference range appears to be more reliable. However, any clinically discordant free T4 results should always be repeated and cross-checked in different assay platforms.

3.3.3 Serum Total T3/Free T3

Measurement of T3 is usually only required for evaluation of hyperthyroid state in pregnancy. Similar to total T4, total T3 is also increased in pregnancy secondary to increase in TBG concentration. Gestational age-based modifications of nonpregnant reference range as described in the earlier section for total T4, should also be used for total T3 levels in pregnancy [28, 36]. However, total T3 level was found to be significantly higher in the third trimester, in comparison to second trimester indicating a progressive rise even in later half of the pregnancy [37]. Free T3 concentrations measured by indirect immunoassays are less robust and inaccuracies due to interferences are commonly encountered. More reliable direct assays like equilibrium dialysis and LC/MS are very costly and practically not available except in some research institutes. Total T3 with pregnancy adjusted reference range is mainly used for evaluation of maternal T3 status in day-to-day clinical practice.

Case Scenario 1

A 24-year-old pregnant lady is admitted to antenatal ward due to severe nausea and vomiting. She is currently in her 12th week of gestation. She gives a history of progressively increasing severity of nausea, vomiting, tiredness, and palpitations for the last 3 weeks and she has lost 2 kgs of body weight. Her pulse rate is 86/min and regular in rhythm and BP is 110/70. There is no neck swelling or any eye changes. Her laboratory results showed: TSH 0.2 mIU/L (0.1–4 mIU/L), FT4 1.7 ng/dl (0.8–1.8 ng/dl), total T4 14 μg/dl (5–12 μg/dl), LFT–normal. Her prepregnancy thyroid function test was normal. What will be her management?

Answer: Reassurance and no medical treatment is needed. The total T4 is within the reference range after correcting for the gestational age.

3.3.4 Thyroid Autoantibodies

Anti-TPO and anti-Tg antibodies are mainly used for the assessment of thyroid autoimmunity in pregnancy. Thyroid autoimmunity can affect fetal and maternal outcomes and plays a pivotal role in deciding the need for levothyroxine treatment especially in subclinical hypothyroidism. Although Anti-TPO antibodies are mostly used by studies to detect thyroid autoimmunity and its clinical outcome, testing for only anti-TPO antibody is likely to miss the diagnosis of isolated anti-Tg antibody positivity in a small cohort of patients. More importantly, serum TSH was reported to be significantly higher in these patients with isolated positive anti-Tg antibody [38]. Dietary iodine intake and ethnicity can also affect thyroid antibody positivity in pregnancy [39]. Thyroid antibody positivity is also reported to decrease with increasing gestational age [40]. In a recent meta-analysis, Korevaar et al. reported that cut-offs used by assays to define anti-TPO antibody positivity were too high [41]. At the population level, the current cut-off will miss around 29% pregnant women, whose antibody concentration is high enough to affect maternal thyroid function and pregnancy outcome. One of the major problems with the analysis of these antibodies is the use of a wide range of cut-offs by different assay methods and the lack of concordance between the assay results [42].

Measurement of TRAb is mainly advised for the diagnosis of maternal Graves' disease and its monitoring during pregnancy and to assess the risk of development of fetal thyrotoxicosis. TRAb can be subdivided functionally according to its action on TSH receptors-stimulating (TSAbs), blocking (TBAbs), and neutral (N-TRAbs) [43]. TSAbs is the antibody responsible for the pathogenesis of Graves' diseases and rarely fetal thyrotoxicosis. On the other hand, transplacental passage of TBAbs can lead to transient fetal hypothyroidism. Commercially available assay can only measure the total TRAbs and not its functional subtypes. Cyclic AMP-based "bioassay" can differentiate between TSAbs and TBAbs, but it is not widely available except in research settings [44].

Case scenario 2

A 32-year-old lady at 5 weeks of pregnancy presented for evaluation. She has history of infertility. She does not have past history of thyroid disease. Her TSH was 3.9 mIU/L. What to do next?

Answer: Anti-TPO/Anti-Tg antibody should be advised to decide whether to start levothyroxine or not. The threshold for treatment with levothyroxine depends upon the TSH and thyroid autoimmunity status.

3.4 Approach to Thyroid Disorders in Pregnancy

In most of the guidelines, TSH is advised as the first screening test for thyroid disorders in pregnancy. If the TSH value is higher than the population and trimester-specific cut-off, then serum T4 (free or total) measurement should be done. The diagnosis of overt or subclinical hypothyroidism can be made depending upon the T4 concentration of below or within the reference range respectively. Evaluation of thyroid autoimmunity status (anti-TPO Antibody and/or anti-Tg antibody) is relevant specifically in subclinical hypothyroidism cases as the threshold of initiation of levothyroxine therapy depends upon the TSH level and autoimmunity status [3].

If the TSH value is below the population and trimester-specific cut-off, then serum T4 (free or total) and total T3 should be measured [36]. Suppressed TSH with high T3 or T4 is defined as overt hyperthyroidism and on the other hand if T3 and T4 levels are normal, a diagnosis of subclinical hypothyroidism is made. The two most common differentials of hyperthyroidism in pregnancy are gestational thyrotoxicosis and Graves' disease. A positive TRAb titer can confirm the diagnosis of Graves's disease. Apart from clinical cues, a higher T3/T4 ratio can also be a surrogate marker in favor of diagnosis of Graves' disease.

Case scenario 3

A 27-year-old lady at 18 weeks of gestation was prescribed the tablet Carbimazole for a biochemical profile that showed her TSH to be suppressed (0.01 mIU/L) with elevated total T4 18 μg/dl (5–12 μg/dl). She has mild diffuse goiter with palpitations and is otherwise normal. She has come for a second opinion.

Answer: Tablet Carbimazole can be withheld for the time being and reinitiated after TRAb testing in maternal hyperthyroidism.

A normal TSH value with a low free T4 level is diagnosed as isolated maternal hypothyroxinemia. In patients with normal TSH and positive thyroid antibody (euthyroid-positive autoimmunity), serial measurement of TSH during pregnancy is recommended [3].

The laboratory cut-offs for diagnosing common thyroid disorders of pregnancy are given in Table 3.3.

A pragmatic flow chart for the diagnosis of common thyroid disorders in pregnancy is depicted in Fig. 3.1.

Table 3.3 Diagnostic cut-off for common pregnancy-specific thyroid disorders (As per ATA guideline, 2017) [3]

Diagnosis	Criteria
Maternal hypothyroidism	TSH more than the upper limit of the pregnancy and population-specific reference range (>4.0 mU/L where pregnancy-specific reference range is not available or reduction of 0.5 mU/L from nonpregnant reference range)
Maternal overt hypothyroidism	High TSH (as described above) level with fT4 or TT4 level below the lower limit of pregnancy-specific reference range
Maternal subclinical hypothyroidism	High TSH (as described above) level with fT4 or TT4 level within pregnancy-specific reference range
Isolated hypothyroxinemia	Low fT4 concentration as per the pregnancy and population-specific reference range with normal maternal TSH level
Thyrotoxicosis in pregnancy	Maternal TSH level less than lower limit of pregnancy-specific reference range (<0.1 mU/L where pregnancy-specific reference range is not available or reduction of 0.4 mU/L from nonpregnant reference range in the first trimester)
Overt thyrotoxicosis in pregnancy	Subnormal TSH (as defined above) with T3/T4 level above the pregnancy-specific reference range
Subclinical thyrotoxicosis in pregnancy	Subnormal TSH (as defined above) with T3/T4 level within the pregnancy-specific reference range

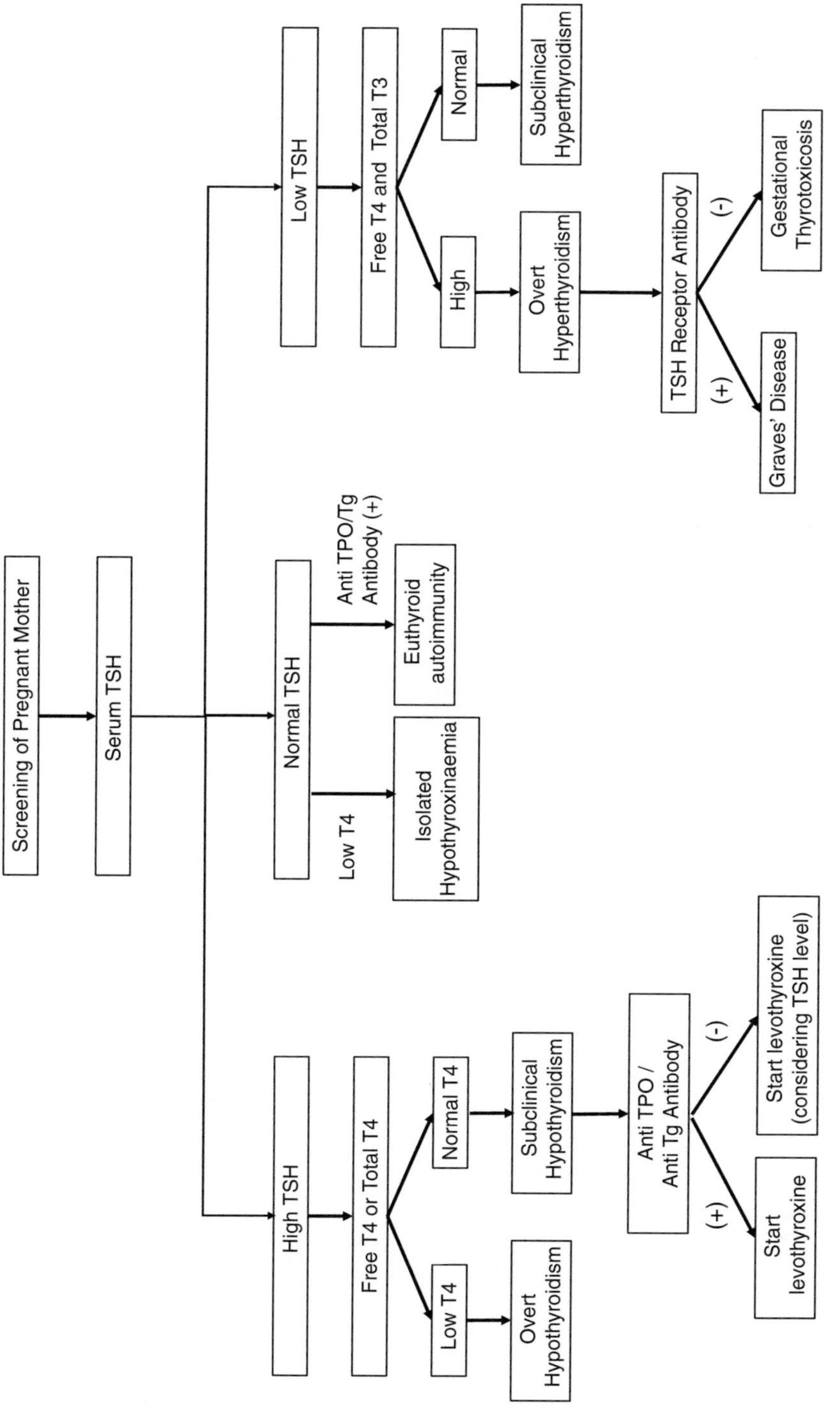

Fig. 3.1 A pragmatic approach to common thyroid disorders during pregnancy. *Anti-Tg* Anti-Thyroglobulin; *Anti-TPO* Anti-Thyroid Peroxidase; *T3* triiodothyronine; *T4* tetraiodothyronine; *TSH* Thyroid Stimulating Hormone

Key Messages

- Screening of pregnant mothers in early pregnancy to diagnose thyroid disorders is needed specifically in those with high-risk factors.
- The total T3 and T4 levels should be interpreted according to gestational age due to increased TBG levels.
- TSH value should be interpreted ideally according to the population and trimester-specific cut-offs.

References

1. Lee SY, Pearce EN. Assessment and treatment of thyroid disorders in pregnancy and the postpartum period. Nat Rev Endocrinol. 2022;18:158–71.
2. Tsakiridis I, Giouleka S, Kourtis A, Mamopoulos A, Athanasiadis A, Dagklis T. Thyroid disease in pregnancy: a descriptive review of guidelines. Obstet Gynecol Surv. 2022;77:45–62.
3. Alexander EK, Pearce EN, Brent GA, Brown RS, Chen H, Dosiou C, et al. Guidelines of the American Thyroid Association for the diagnosis and Management of Thyroid Disease during Pregnancy and the postpartum. Thyroid. 2017;27:315–89.
4. Dong AC, Stagnaro-Green A. Differences in diagnostic criteria mask the true prevalence of thyroid disease in pregnancy: a systematic review and meta-analysis. Thyroid. 2019;29:278–89.
5. Taylor PN, Albrecht D, Scholz A, Gutierrez-Buey G, Lazarus JH, Dayan CM, et al. Global epidemiology of hyperthyroidism and hypothyroidism. Nat Rev Endocrinol. 2018;14:301–16.
6. Vila L, Velasco I, González S, Morales F, Sánchez E, Lailla JM, et al. Detection of thyroid dysfunction in pregnant women: universal screening is justified. Endocrinol Nutr. 2012;59:547–60.
7. Negro R, Beck-Peccoz P, Chiovato L, Garofalo P, Guglielmi R, Papini E, et al. Hyperthyroidism and pregnancy. An Italian thyroid association (AIT) and Italian Association of Clinical Endocrinologists (AME) joint statement for clinical practice. J Endocrinol Investig. 2011;34:225–31.
8. Thyroid Disease in Pregnancy. ACOG practice bulletin, number 223. Obstet Gynecol. 2020;135:e261–74.
9. National_Guidelines_for_Screening_of_Hypothyroidism_during_Pregnancy.pdf [Internet]. [cited 2021 Nov 17]. Available from: http://www.nrhmorissa.gov.in/writereaddata/Upload/Documents/National_Guidelines_for_Screening_of_Hypothyroidism_during_Pregnancy.pdf
10. Sgarbi JA, Teixeira PFS, Maciel LMZ, Mazeto GMFS, Vaisman M, Montenegro Junior RM, et al. The Brazilian consensus for the clinical approach and treatment of subclinical hypothyroidism in adults: recommendations of the thyroid Department of the Brazilian Society of endocrinology and metabolism. Arq Bras Endocrinol Metabol. 2013;57:166–83.
11. Lazarus JH, Bestwick JP, Channon S, Paradice R, Maina A, Rees R, et al. Antenatal thyroid screening and childhood cognitive function. N Engl J Med. 2012;366:493–501.
12. Korevaar TIM, Muetzel R, Medici M, Chaker L, Jaddoe VWV, de Rijke YB, et al. Association of maternal thyroid function during early pregnancy with offspring IQ and brain morphology in childhood: a population-based prospective cohort study. Lancet Diabetes Endocrinol. 2016;4:35–43.
13. Wilson JMG, Jungner G, Organization WH. Principles and practice of screening for disease [internet]. World Health Organization; 1968. Available from: https://apps.who.int/iris/handle/10665/37650
14. Taylor PN, Zouras S, Min T, Nagarahaj K, Lazarus JH, Okosieme O. Thyroid screening in early pregnancy: pros and cons. Front Endocrinol (Lausanne). 2018;9:626.

15. Stagnaro-Green A, Dong A, Stephenson MD. Universal screening for thyroid disease during pregnancy should be performed. Best Pract Res Clin Endocrinol Metab. 2020;34:101320.
16. Dosiou C, Barnes J, Schwartz A, Negro R, Crapo L, Stagnaro-Green A. Cost-effectiveness of universal and risk-based screening for autoimmune thyroid disease in pregnant women. J Clin Endocrinol Metab. 2012;97:1536–46.
17. Donnay Candil S, Balsa Barro JA, Álvarez Hernández J, Crespo Palomo C, Pérez-Alcántara F, Polanco Sánchez C. Cost-effectiveness analysis of universal screening for thyroid disease in pregnant women in Spain. Endocrinol Nutr. 2015;62:322–30.
18. Azizi F, Mehran L, Amouzegar A, Alamdari S, Subetki I, Saadat N, et al. Prevalent practices of thyroid diseases during pregnancy among endocrinologists, internists and general practitioners. Int J Endocrinol Metab. 2016;14:e29601.
19. Koren R, Wiener Y, Or K, Benbassat CA, Koren S. Thyroid disease in pregnancy: a clinical survey among endocrinologists, gynecologists, and obstetricians in Israel. Isr Med Assoc J. 2018;20:167–71.
20. Salmeen KE, Block-Kurbisch IJ. Chapter 4–thyroid physiology during pregnancy, postpartum, and lactation. In: Kovacs CS, Deal CL, editors. Maternal-fetal and neonatal endocrinology [internet]. Academic Press; 2020. p. 53–60. Available from: https://www.sciencedirect.com/science/article/pii/B9780128148235000040.
21. Dashe JS, Casey BM, Wells CE, McIntire DD, Byrd EW, Leveno KJ, et al. Thyroid-stimulating hormone in singleton and twin pregnancy: importance of gestational age-specific reference ranges. Obstet Gynecol. 2005;106:753–7.
22. Lambert-Messerlian G, McClain M, Haddow JE, Palomaki GE, Canick JA, Cleary-Goldman J, et al. First- and second-trimester thyroid hormone reference data in pregnant women: a FaSTER (first- and second-trimester evaluation of risk for aneuploidy) research consortium study. Am J Obstet Gynecol. 2008;199(62):e1–6.
23. Korevaar TIM, Steegers EAP, Pop VJ, Broeren MA, Chaker L, de Rijke YB, et al. Thyroid autoimmunity impairs the thyroidal response to human chorionic gonadotropin: two population-based prospective cohort studies. J Clin Endocrinol Metab. 2017;102:69–77.
24. Glinoer D. The regulation of thyroid function during normal pregnancy: importance of the iodine nutrition status. Best Pract Res Clin Endocrinol Metab. 2004;18:133–52.
25. La'ulu SL, Roberts WL. Ethnic differences in first-trimester thyroid reference intervals. Clin Chem. 2011;57:913–5.
26. Baloch Z, Carayon P, Conte-Devolx B, Demers LM, Feldt-Rasmussen U, Henry J-F, et al. Laboratory medicine practice guidelines. Laboratory support for the diagnosis and monitoring of thyroid disease. Thyroid. 2003;13:3–126.
27. Hattori N, Aisaka K, Chihara K, Shimatsu A. Current thyrotropin immunoassays recognize macro-thyrotropin leading to Hyperthyrotropinemia in females of reproductive age. Thyroid. 2018;28:1252–60.
28. Weeke J, Dybkjaer L, Granlie K, Eskjaer Jensen S, Kjaerulff E, Laurberg P, et al. A longitudinal study of serum TSH, and total and free iodothyronines during normal pregnancy. Acta Endocrinol. 1982;101:531–7.
29. La'ulu SL, Roberts WL. Second-trimester reference intervals for thyroid tests: the role of ethnicity. Clin Chem. 2007;53:1658–64.
30. Lee RH, Spencer CA, Mestman JH, Miller EA, Petrovic I, Braverman LE, et al. Free T4 immunoassays are flawed during pregnancy. Am J Obstet Gynecol. 2009;200(260):e1–6.
31. Stockigt JR, Lim C-F. Medications that distort in vitro tests of thyroid function, with particular reference to estimates of serum free thyroxine. Best Pract Res Clin Endocrinol Metab. 2009;23:753–67.
32. Zhang Y, Wang R, Dong Y, Huang G, Ji B, Wang Q. Assessment of biotin interference in thyroid function tests. Medicine (Baltimore). 2020;99:e19232.
33. Kahric-Janicic N, Soldin SJ, Soldin OP, West T, Gu J, Jonklaas J. Tandem mass spectrometry improves the accuracy of free thyroxine measurements during pregnancy. Thyroid. 2007;17:303–11.

34. Levie D, Korevaar TIM, Bath SC, Dalmau-Bueno A, Murcia M, Espada M, et al. Thyroid function in early pregnancy, child IQ, and autistic traits: a meta-analysis of individual participant data. J Clin Endocrinol Metab. 2018;103:2967–79.
35. Korevaar TIM, Chaker L, Medici M, de Rijke YB, Jaddoe VWV, Steegers EAP, et al. Maternal total T4 during the first half of pregnancy: physiologic aspects and the risk of adverse outcomes in comparison with free T4. Clin Endocrinol. 2016;85:757–63.
36. Lee SY, Pearce EN. Testing, monitoring, and treatment of thyroid dysfunction in pregnancy. J Clin Endocrinol Metab. 2021;106:883–92.
37. Soldin OP, Tractenberg RE, Hollowell JG, Jonklaas J, Janicic N, Soldin SJ. Trimester-specific changes in maternal thyroid hormone, thyrotropin, and thyroglobulin concentrations during gestation: trends and associations across trimesters in iodine sufficiency. Thyroid. 2004;14:1084–90.
38. Unuane D, Velkeniers B, Anckaert E, Schiettecatte J, Tournaye H, Haentjens P, et al. Thyroglobulin autoantibodies: is there any added value in the detection of thyroid autoimmunity in women consulting for fertility treatment? Thyroid. 2013;23:1022–8.
39. Shi X, Han C, Li C, Mao J, Wang W, Xie X, et al. Optimal and safe upper limits of iodine intake for early pregnancy in iodine-sufficient regions: a cross-sectional study of 7190 pregnant women in China. J Clin Endocrinol Metab. 2015;100:1630–8.
40. Ekinci EI, Chiu W-L, Lu ZX, Sikaris K, Churilov L, Bittar I, et al. A longitudinal study of thyroid autoantibodies in pregnancy: the importance of test timing. Clin Endocrinol. 2015;82:604–10.
41. Korevaar TIM, Pop VJ, Chaker L, Goddijn M, de Rijke YB, Bisschop PH, et al. Dose dependency and a functional cutoff for TPO-antibody positivity during pregnancy. J Clin Endocrinol Metab. 2018;103:778–89.
42. McNeil AR, Stanford PE. Reporting thyroid function tests in pregnancy. Clin Biochem Rev. 2015;36:109–26.
43. Li C, Zhou J, Huang Z, Pan X, Leung W, Chen L, et al. The clinical value and variation of Antithyroid antibodies during pregnancy. Dis Markers. 2020;2020:8871951.
44. Abeillon-du Payrat J, Chikh K, Bossard N, Bretones P, Gaucherand P, Claris O, et al. Predictive value of maternal second-generation thyroid-binding inhibitory immunoglobulin assay for neonatal autoimmune hyperthyroidism. Eur J Endocrinol. 2014;171:451–60.

Thyroid Autoimmunity and Pregnancy

4

Kalyani Sridharan

4.1 Introduction

Thyroid autoimmunity (TAI) is a common clinical problem during pregnancy [1]. It may or may not be associated with thyroid dysfunction during pregnancy. Presence of anti-thyroid antibodies has been associated with adverse pregnancy outcomes [2]. This association in an individual patient is further modified by several factors like the degree and duration of thyroid dysfunction and iodine deficiency. Treatment aimed at optimising maternal and foetal outcomes with levothyroxine (LT4) has been studied with varying results [2]. This chapter discusses the extent of the problem, summarises the available evidence on the various treatment modalities and contextualises the problem with the help of a few case scenarios.

4.2 Prevalence of Thyroid Autoantibodies during Pregnancy

TAI is most commonly mediated by three antibodies: anti-thyroid peroxidase antibodies (TPO-Ab), anti-thyroglobulin antibodies (Tg-Ab) and thyrotropin receptor antibodies (TRAb). Most studies assessing for prevalence of thyroid antibodies during pregnancy have used only TPO-Ab. Globally, the prevalence of TPO-Ab in unselected pregnant women ranges between 2 and 17% [1]. Studies in India have shown the prevalence of TPO-Ab in unselected pregnant women to range between 10% and 19% [3–6] and Tg-Ab to be 14% [4]. The prevalence of thyroid autoantibodies increases as the level of thyrotropin (TSH) increases such that in pregnant patients with elevated TSH levels the prevalence of TPO-Ab ranges between 30 and 60% [1]. The prevalence of TAI is also more in pregnant women with a history of

K. Sridharan (✉)
All India Institute of Medical Sciences, Rishikesh, Uttarakhand, India

H. Sagili et al. (eds.), *Thyroid Disease in Pregnancy - A Guide to Clinical Management*, https://doi.org/10.1007/978-981-99-5423-0_4

recurrent pregnancy loss [7, 8]. In addition to pregnant women, among non-pregnant women, thyroid autoantibodies are associated with female factor infertility and polycystic ovarian syndrome [1].

4.3 TAI and Reproductive Pathophysiology

Several theories explaining the association between TAI and pregnancy complications have been put forward although, most of them remain hypothetical. Thyroid hormone (TH) receptors as well as transporters are present in reproductive tissues like ovary, endometrium, uterus, early embryo and placenta [9]. TH acting synergistically with follicle-stimulating hormone (FSH) promotes granulosa cell proliferation, inhibits its apoptosis and increases the expression of matrix metalloproteinases on placental trophoblasts [9]. Recent evidence also suggests the importance of TH signalling during embryo implantation and early pregnancy [10]. Women with TPO-Ab positivity have been shown to have abnormal uterine artery pulsatility indices and placental features of maternal vascular malperfusion as compared to women without TPO-Ab [11]. In a recent study for the first time, thyroid peroxidase enzyme has been isolated by immunohistochemistry on human granulosa cumulus cells lending credence to the possibility of a direct pathophysiological effect [12]. In the same fashion that TH affects reproductive tissues, reproductive hormones most notably human chorionic gonadotropin (hCG) also affect the TH. The linear relationship between hCG and thyroxine and the inverse relationship between hCG and TSH is blunted in women with TPO-Ab positivity [13]. However, the mechanisms underlying the above associations are not completely clear.

Three theories have been proposed to explain the association between thyroid autoantibodies and adverse pregnancy outcomes. One is that TAI is a mere marker of a generalised autoimmune phenomenon and the pregnancy complications are the result of a hostile uterine microenvironment. Another hypothesis is that the TAI causes a state of impaired TH reserve and since TH is necessary for implantation, this insufficiency is probably associated with pregnancy loss. A third hypothesis is that the thyroid autoantibodies are directly pathogenic to the developing embryo [2, 14]. A recent study proposes a unifying pathophysiological model to reconcile the above three independent theories. According to the proposed model in the initial stages of TAI, the response of TH to hCG remains intact but the TPO-Ab act at the granulosa cells directly creating a hostile local immune response. At the later stages of TAI, the response of TH to hCG becomes blunted resulting in insufficient TH levels at the reproductive tissues impairing implantation, in addition to the local immune response [2]. The levels of thyroid autoantibodies decrease during pregnancy with highest levels seen in the first trimester [15]. In spite of this decline, pregnant women with TAI show a progressive increase in TSH levels throughout gestation [15, 16]. This emphasises the decreased ability of the thyroid gland to adapt to the increased TH requirements during pregnancy in women with TAI.

4.4 TAI and Maternal Thyroid Dysfunction during Pregnancy and Post-Partum

Pregnant women with TAI have a higher risk of developing thyroid dysfunction during pregnancy and in the post-partum period. In a prospective cohort study, which followed 87 euthyroid pregnant women with TPO-Ab positivity through gestation, 16% developed a TSH level of more than 4 mIU/ml at delivery [15]. Euthyroid women with TAI in the first trimester had higher TSH levels as compared to women without TAI. It is therefore imperative to monitor euthyroid women with TAI with TSH every 4 weeks [1]. Presence of TAI during pregnancy also predicts future development of thyroid disease. The risk was increased fourfold in pregnant women with TPO-Ab positivity who were euthyroid as compared to eightfold if the women were both TPO-Ab positive and hypothyroid [17]. Several studies have documented an association between TAI and post-partum thyroiditis (PPT) [8, 18]. In a large prospective study, PPT occurred at a mean time of 6 weeks post-partum. Performing a thyroid function at 6 weeks post-partum would be appropriate in the timely diagnosis of PPT.

4.5 TAI and Adverse Pregnancy Outcomes

There is accumulating evidence in the past decade that TAI is associated with both maternal and foetal adverse outcomes.

Adverse Maternal Outcomes

1. *Pregnancy loss:*

Three meta-analyses showed a significant association between TAI and spontaneous pregnancy loss [8, 19, 20]. The studies showed that there was more than tripling of the odds of miscarriage and doubling of the odds of recurrent miscarriage in women with TAI. These women were also older and had higher TSH levels. Overall, the data for association with TAI is more robust for sporadic pregnancy loss as compared to recurrent pregnancy loss as the latter more often has other causes rather than endocrine dysfunction. More recent prospective data also support the increased risk of miscarriage with TAI and also show that this risk is more in the patients with TAI and subclinical hypothyroidism compared to those with TAI and euthyroidism [21]. Therefore to summarise, the evidence for association between TAI and pregnancy loss is robust although this does not prove causality.

2. *Premature Birth:*

Although small observational data had conflicting results on the association between TAI and prematurity, two large meta-analyses demonstrated a clear association between the two [20, 22]. A recent individual participant data meta-analysis involving 47,045 women showed that TPO-Ab but not Tg-Ab was associated with increased risk of pre-term (< 37 weeks gestational age) and very pre-term birth (<32 weeks gestational age) and this risk was modified by TSH concentration [23].

3. *Placental abruption:*

With regard to the association between TAI and placental abruption, the evidence is less robust. One prospective study showed threefold increased risk of placental abruption in women with TAI as compared to women without TAI [24]. More studies are needed to confirm or refute this association.

4. *Pre-eclampsia:*

There are only a few studies that studied association between TAI and pre-eclampsia. A meta-analysis showed no association although it included only a single study [8]. A prospective study with 600 patients showed an association between TAI and pre-eclampsia but they found that this association was significant only in the subgroup with thyroid dysfunction [25].

5. *Gestational diabetes:*

There is more evidence accumulating confirming the association between TAI and gestational diabetes mellitus (GDM). A meta-analysis done in 2011 which included only one study showed no association between TAI and GDM [8]. However, several prospective studies done after that and a more recent meta-analysis of those studies with around 34,000 patients showed a significant association between GDM and TAI with or without thyroid dysfunction [26].

6. *Premature rupture of membranes and polyhydramnios:*

Some studies demonstrated an association between TAI and pre-term premature rupture of membranes [27] and polyhydramnios [18] while others did not [8]. In the absence of large prospective studies, it is not possible to conclude for or against the association.

7. *Post-natal depression:*

TAI has been frequently associated with post-natal mood changes, depression and alexithymia. A recent large systematic review that did a qualitative analysis on the effect of thyroid function and TAI on post-partum patient outcomes conclude that unlike thyroid dysfunction, thyroid autoantibodies were more consistently associated with post-partum mood disturbances [28].

Adverse Foetal Outcomes

1. *Neurocognitive disability:*

Several studies have studied an association between TAI in the mother and neurocognitive outcomes in the child. A prospective study that followed 97 mother-child pairs demonstrated that children born to mothers with TAI had lower perceptual performance and motor scores at 5.5 years of age, although there was no association with neurodevelopment outcomes [29]. Another prospective study showed an association of maternal TAI with development of sensorineural hearing loss (SNHL) in the child at 8 years of age [30]. A study in the same cohort showed that in women with TAI, the child intelligent quotient (IQ) scores were modestly lower at 4 years of age but not at 7 years of age. The authors speculate that this effect could be mediated by SNHL [31]. A recent large cohort study from Greece also confirmed the finding of increased risk of decreased perceptual and motor ability in children at 4 years of age [32]. A large cohort study of 3000 children showed maternal TPO-Ab positivity to be associated with attention deficit hyperactivity syndrome in children but did not predict neurodevelopmental outcomes [33].

2. *Low birthweight:*

The association between maternal TAI and birthweight is not clear. While one study showed a positive association [34], another did not show any such association [35].

4.6 TAI and Infertility and Assisted Reproduction

TAI has been shown to be associated with female factor infertility and also affects the response to therapy with clomiphene citrate in some studies [36, 37]. Two meta-analyses showed that euthyroid women with TAI undergoing in vitro fertilisation (IVF) had a greater miscarriage rate but no difference in clinical pregnancy rate when compared to women without TAI [38, 39]. In contrast, another recent meta-analysis of euthyroid women with TAI undergoing IVF or intra-cytoplasmic sperm injection (ICSI) showed no difference in clinical pregnancy rates, miscarriage rate or live birth rates when compared to euthyroid women undergoing IVF/ICSI without TAI [40].

Case scenario 1

A 30-year-old woman with 8 weeks of gestation has tested positive for TPO-Ab but is euthyroid on thyroid function tests. She is worried about the risk to her and her baby and comes to you for advice regarding maternal and foetal risk. What will you tell her?

Answer: Published literature show an increased risk of certain maternal and foetal outcomes with thyroid autoimmunity like pregnancy loss, pre-term birth, gestational diabetes, thyroid dysfunction, post-partum thyroiditis and post-partum mood disturbances. Evidence is equivocal or uncertain regarding association with other outcomes like placental abruption, pre-eclampsia or polyhydramnios. Of the foetal outcomes, evidence for association with neuro-cognitive disability is lacking while there is some association with ADHD.

4.7 Treatment of TAI

Treatment modalities that have been tried in TAI include LT4, selenium, oral steroids and intravenous immunoglobulins (IVIG). The following discussion summarises the evidence for use of these modalities to date and the current recommendations of the American Thyroid Association (ATA).

4.7.1 Levothyroxine

By far, Levothyroxine (LT4) is the most commonly used treatment for TAI with or without thyroid dysfunction in pregnancy in studies. Table 4.1 gives an overview of the current published literature with regard to use of LT4 in various subsets of pregnant patients with TAI and summarises the ATA 2017 recommendations on the same. The evidence is best and unequivocal for LT4 treatment in women with overt hypothyroidism during pregnancy irrespective of the antibody status. In pregnant women with TAI and subclinical hypothyroidism (SCH) or euthyroidism, although association with adverse maternal and some foetal events is established well, results of treatment with LT4 have so far been disappointing. Evidence accumulated after the 2017 ATA recommendations, especially the TABLET trial and a small Iranian randomised controlled trial (RCT) failed to demonstrate benefit with LT4 even when started pre-conception [41, 42]. Similarly, benefit of LT4 in euthyroid pregnant women planning artificial reproductive techniques (ART) is also lacking. The study by Wang et al. [43], in fact, calls for a change in the current ATA weak recommendation on considering LT4 therapy in women with TAI undergoing ART. Studies examining LT4 therapy in pregnant women with SCH to prevent child-adverse neurocognitive development have also not shown positive results, although it could be argued that LT4 therapy was not started early in the first trimester [44, 45].

Case scenario 2

A 33-year-old primi gravida presents at 12 weeks gestation with a TSH of 6.5 uIU/ml (upper limit of lab cut-off is 4.0 uIU/ml) and positive anti-TPO antibodies. How do you manage her?

Answer: She will require treatment with levothyroxine (LT4 50 µg once daily) and monitoring with thyroid function to a TSH target of less than 2.5 uIU/ml.

Table 4.1 Overview of evidence summary on the use of LT4 for TAI during pregnancy

Patient cohort	Summary of ATA 2017 recommendations [1]	Summary of studies after ATA 2017	Remarks
Euthyroid pregnant women with TAI	Insufficient evidence to recommend for or against treating with LT4 to prevent pre-term birth or pregnancy loss	A meta-analysis showed no association between LT4 treatment and live birth rate [46]	Evidence is accumulating towards not treating with LT4
Euthyroid TAI pregnant women with past recurrent miscarriages	Administration of LT4 may be considered given its potential benefits in comparison with its minimal risk	A double-blind, placebo-controlled trial to investigate whether levothyroxine treatment would increase live birth rates among euthyroid women who had thyroid peroxidase antibodies and a history of miscarriage or infertility showed no difference in live birth rate, miscarriage rate or pregnancy rate [41]	Newer evidence does not support this recommendation to treat with LT4
Euthyroid women with TAI and infertility	Insufficient evidence to determine if LT4 therapy improvesfertilityinnon-pregnant,thyroidautoantibody-positive euthyroid women who are attempting natural conception	A double-blind, placebo-controlled trial to investigate whether levothyroxine treatment would increase live birth rates among euthyroid women who had thyroid peroxidase antibodies and a history of miscarriage or infertility showed no difference in live birth rate, miscarriage rate or pregnancy rate [41]	Only one trial showed no effect of treatment; further studies needed

(continued)

Table 4.1 (continued)

Patient cohort	Summary of ATA 2017 recommendations [1]	Summary of studies after ATA 2017	Remarks
Pregnant TAI women with subclinical hypothyroidism (SCH)	(a) LT4 therapy is recommended for – TPOAb-positive women with a TSH > pregnancy-specific reference range – TPOAb-negative women with a TSH >10.0 mU/L (b) LT4 therapy may be considered for – TPOAb-positive women with TSH >2.5 mU/L and < upper limit of the pregnancy-specific reference range. – TPOAb-negative women with TSH > pregnancy-specific reference range and < 10.0 mU/L (c) LT4 therapy is not recommended for- TPOAb-negative women with a normal TSH (TSH within the pregnancy-specific reference range)	None	No new evidence after ATA 2017 to the contrary
TAI women post-ART	Insufficient evidence to determine whether LT4 therapy improves the success of pregnancy following ART in TPOAb-positive euthyroid women but administration of LT4 may be considered given its potential benefits in comparison to its minimal risk"	The POSTAL trial RCT showed no difference in live birth rate, miscarriage rate or pregnancy rate in LT4 treated vs non-treated [43]	Evidence is accumulating towards not treating with LT4

ATA American Thyroid Association; *TAI* Thyroid autoimmunity; *RCT* Randomised controlled trial; *LT4* Levothyroxine; *TSH* Thyroid stimulating hormone; *TPO-Ab* Anti-thyroid peroxidase antibodies

4.7.2 Selenium

In the thyroid cells, glutathione peroxidase enzyme requires selenium as a cofactor. Selenium deficiency, therefore, has been shown to be associated with thyroid cell necrosis [47]. Evidence in non-pregnant patients that selenium supplementation can decrease thyroid inflammation and TPO-Ab levels is conflicting [48–50]. One RCT showed a reduction in post-partum thyroid disease and TPO-Ab titers in pregnant patients supplemented with selenomethionine [51]. However, the study did not adjust for iodine status in the cohort. This finding could not be replicated in another study conducted in mildly iodine-deficient pregnant women [52] while another study showed that selenium supplementation could increase the risk of type 2 diabetes mellitus [53]. Therefore, current ATA guidelines do not recommend selenium supplementation in pregnant women.

4.7.3 Oral Steroids and IVIG

Oral steroids and IVIG have been tried during pregnancy for TAI although most of the studies have been small resulting in overall insufficient evidence to recommend either therapy. Two small RCTs studied use of oral steroids in pregnant women with TAI undergoing ART and concluded that this resulted in improved pregnancy rates with or without reduced miscarriage rates [54, 55]. Three small non-randomised studies have reported on the use of IVIG in pregnant women with TAI [56–58]. Two of these studies reported improved live birth rates with IVIG [56, 57], while one study found no benefit when compared to LT4 supplementation [58].

4.8 Screening and Monitoring in Women with TAI during Pregnancy and Post-partum

Although, as discussed earlier, most studies have shown an association of TAI with adverse pregnancy outcomes and some foetal outcomes, there is no consensus on whether LT4 supplementation improves maternal or foetal outcomes. In fact, recent RCTs failed to show benefit of LT4 even when started before conception [41]. Hence, current guidelines do not recommend universal screening for TAI [1, 14].

Euthyroid pregnant women with TAI are at increased risk of developing hypothyroidism. Therefore, ATA recommends that such women be monitored with TSH levels at the time of confirmation of pregnancy and then every 4 weeks till mid-gestation [1].

Case scenario 3

A pregnant woman presents at 12 weeks with positive anti-TPO antibodies and a TSH of 2.3 uIU/ml. How will you treat and monitor her during pregnancy?

Answer: The ATA 2017 guidelines conclude that the evidence to treat euthyroid women with thyroid autoimmunity is insufficient. However, more recent RCTs show no benefit in treatment even when started before conception. Even in previous studies benefit of treatment (when seen) was only if started early in gestation not later. Therefore, in the given case, benefit of treatment with LT4 is less likely. However, the risk and benefits should be explained to patient and a shared decision-making would be in the best patient's interest. Since there is evidence that thyroid dysfunction may progress during pregnancy in women with TAI, the patient should be monitored with thyroid function tests throughout pregnancy.

Key Messages

- TAI is a commonly encountered problem in pregnancy.
- There is moderately strong evidence of association of TAI with adverse maternal outcomes like pregnancy loss, pre-term birth, gestational diabetes, post-partum thyroiditis and post-partum mood disturbances; while evidence of association with other pregnancy outcomes like placental abruption, pre-eclampsia and polyhydramnios is uncertain.
- Association of TAI with adverse foetal outcomes exists for ADHD and sensorineural hearing loss while no such association could be demonstrated for neurocognitive disability.
- Putative hypotheses regarding adverse outcomes with TAI include a generalised autoimmune phenomenon with hostile uterine microenvironment, a decreased thyroid hormone reserve or a direct pathogenicity of the TAI to the developing embryo.
- Pregnant women with TAI are at risk of developing thyroid dysfunction during the course of pregnancy so require frequent monitoring of thyroid function during pregnancy.
- Treatment for TAI has been tried with LT4, oral steroids, IVIG and selenium although most studies are with LT4.
- Present evidence supports treating pregnant women with TAI and overt or subclinical hypothyroidism with LT4 while there is no evidence of improved maternal or foetal outcomes in treating euthyroid women with TAI.

Conflict of interest Nil.

Funding Nil.

References

1. Alexander EK, Pearce EN, Brent GA, Brown RS, Chen H, Dosiou C, et al. 2017 guidelines of the American Thyroid Association for the diagnosis and Management of Thyroid Disease during Pregnancy and the postpartum. Thyroid. 2017;27:315–89.
2. Dosiou C. Thyroid and fertility: recent advances. Thyroid. 2020;30:479–86.
3. Rajput R, Yadav T, Seth S, Nanda S. Prevalence of thyroid peroxidase antibody and pregnancy outcome in Euthyroid autoimmune positive pregnant women from a tertiary care center in Haryana. Indian J Endocrinol Metab. 2017;21:577–80.
4. Jaiswal N, Melse-Boonstra A, Thomas T, Basavaraj C, Sharma SK, Srinivasan K, et al. High prevalence of maternal hypothyroidism despite adequate iodine status in Indian pregnant women in the first trimester. Thyroid. 2014;24:1419–29.
5. Meena M, Chopra S, Jain V, Aggarwal N. The effect of anti-thyroid peroxidase antibodies on pregnancy outcomes in Euthyroid women. J Clin Diagn Res. 2016;10:QC04–7.
6. Nambiar V, Jagtap VS, Sarathi V, Lila AR, Kamalanathan S, Bandgar TR, et al. Prevalence and impact of thyroid disorders on maternal outcome in Asian-Indian pregnant women. J Thyroid Res. 2011;2011:429097.
7. Lata K, Dutta P, Sridhar S, Rohilla M, Srinivasan A, Prashad GRV, et al. Thyroid autoimmunity and obstetric outcomes in women with recurrent miscarriage: a case-control study. Endocr Connect. 2013;2:118–24.
8. van den Boogaard E, Vissenberg R, Land JA, van Wely M, van der Post JAM, Goddijn M, et al. Significance of (sub)clinical thyroid dysfunction and thyroid autoimmunity before conception and in early pregnancy: a systematic review. Hum Reprod Update. 2011;17:605–19.
9. Vissenberg R, Manders VD, Mastenbroek S, Fliers E, Afink GB, Ris-Stalpers C, et al. Pathophysiological aspects of thyroid hormone disorders/thyroid peroxidase autoantibodies and reproduction. Hum Reprod Update. 2015;21:378–87.
10. Colicchia M, Campagnolo L, Baldini E, Ulisse S, Valensise H, Moretti C. Molecular basis of thyrotropin and thyroid hormone action during implantation and early development. Hum Reprod Update. 2014;20:884–904.
11. Spinillo A, De Maggio I, Ruspini B, Bellingeri C, Cavagnoli C, Giannico S, et al. Placental pathologic features in thyroid autoimmunity. Placenta. 2021;112:66–72.
12. Monteleone P, Faviana P, Artini PG. Thyroid peroxidase identified in human granulosa cells: another piece to the thyroid-ovary puzzle? Gynecol Endocrinol. 2017;33:574–6.
13. Korevaar TIM, Steegers EAP, Pop VJ, Broeren MA, Chaker L, de Rijke YB, et al. Thyroid autoimmunity impairs the thyroidal response to human chorionic gonadotropin: two population-based prospective cohort studies. J Clin Endocrinol Metab. 2017;102:69–77.
14. Dhillon-Smith RK, Coomarasamy A. TPO antibody positivity and adverse pregnancy outcomes. Best Pract Res Clin Endocrinol Metab. 2020;34:101433.
15. Glinoer D, Riahi M, Grün JP, Kinthaert J. Risk of subclinical hypothyroidism in pregnant women with asymptomatic autoimmune thyroid disorders. J Clin Endocrinol Metab. 1994;79:197–204.
16. Negro R, Formoso G, Mangieri T, Pezzarossa A, Dazzi D, Hassan H. Levothyroxine treatment in euthyroid pregnant women with autoimmune thyroid disease: effects on obstetrical complications. J Clin Endocrinol Metab. 2006;91:2587–91.
17. Männistö T, Vääräsmäki M, Pouta A, Hartikainen A-L, Ruokonen A, Surcel H-M, et al. Thyroid dysfunction and autoantibodies during pregnancy as predictive factors of pregnancy complications and maternal morbidity in later life. J Clin Endocrinol Metab. 2010;95:1084–94.
18. Chen X, Jin B, Xia J, Tao X, Huang X, Sun L, et al. Effects of thyroid peroxidase antibody on maternal and neonatal outcomes in pregnant women in an iodine-sufficient area in China. Int J Endocrinol. 2016;2016:6461380.
19. Chen L, Hu R. Thyroid autoimmunity and miscarriage: a meta-analysis. Clin Endocrinol. 2011;74:513–9.

20. Thangaratinam S, Tan A, Knox E, Kilby MD, Franklyn J, Coomarasamy A. Association between thyroid autoantibodies and miscarriage and preterm birth: meta-analysis of evidence. BMJ. 2011;342:d2616.
21. Liu H, Shan Z, Li C, Mao J, Xie X, Wang W, et al. Maternal subclinical hypothyroidism, thyroid autoimmunity, and the risk of miscarriage: a prospective cohort study. Thyroid. 2014;24:1642–9.
22. He X, Wang P, Wang Z, He X, Xu D, Wang B. Thyroid antibodies and risk of preterm delivery: a meta-analysis of prospective cohort studies. Eur J Endocrinol. 2012;167:455–64.
23. Consortium on Thyroid and Pregnancy—Study Group on Preterm Birth, TIM K, Derakhshan A, Taylor PN, Meima M, Chen L, et al. Association of thyroid function test abnormalities and thyroid autoimmunity with preterm birth: a systematic review and meta-analysis. JAMA. 2019;322:632–41.
24. Abbassi-Ghanavati M, Casey BM, Spong CY, McIntire DD, Halvorson LM, Cunningham FG. Pregnancy outcomes in women with thyroid peroxidase antibodies. Obstet Gynecol. 2010;116:381–6.
25. Saki F, Dabbaghmanesh MH, Ghaemi SZ, Forouhari S, Omrani GR, Bakhshayeshkaram M. Thyroid autoimmunity in pregnancy and its influences on maternal and fetal outcome in Iran (a prospective study). Endocr Res. 2015;40:139–45.
26. Luo J, Wang X, Yuan L, Guo L. Association of thyroid disorders with gestational diabetes mellitus: a meta-analysis. Endocrine. 2021;73:550–60.
27. Haddow JE, Cleary-Goldman J, McClain MR, Palomaki GE, Neveux LM, Lambert-Messerlian G, et al. Thyroperoxidase and thyroglobulin antibodies in early pregnancy and preterm delivery. Obstet Gynecol. 2010;116:58–62.
28. Tuzil J, Bartakova J, Watt T, Dolezal T. Health-related quality of life in women with autoimmune thyroid disease during pregnancy and postpartum: systematic review including 321,850 pregnancies. Expert Rev Pharmacoecon Outcomes Res. 2021;21:1–15.
29. Williams FLR, Watson J, Ogston SA, Visser TJ, Hume R, Willatts P. Maternal and umbilical cord levels of T4, FT4, TSH, TPOAb, and TgAb in term infants and neurodevelopmental outcome at 5.5 years. J Clin Endocrinol Metab. 2013;98:829–38.
30. Wasserman EE, Nelson K, Rose NR, Eaton W, Pillion JP, Seaberg E, et al. Maternal thyroid autoantibodies during the third trimester and hearing deficits in children: an epidemiologic assessment. Am J Epidemiol. 2008;167:701–10.
31. Wasserman EE, Pillion JP, Duggan A, Nelson K, Rohde C, Seaberg EC, et al. Childhood IQ, hearing loss, and maternal thyroid autoimmunity in the Baltimore collaborative perinatal project. Pediatr Res. 2012;72:525–30.
32. Kampouri M, Margetaki K, Koutra K, Kyriklaki A, Karakosta P, Anousaki D, et al. Maternal mild thyroid dysfunction and offspring cognitive and motor development from infancy to childhood: the Rhea mother-child cohort study in Crete, Greece. J Epidemiol Community Health. 2021;75:29–35.
33. Ghassabian A, Bongers-Schokking JJ, de Rijke YB, van Mil N, Jaddoe VWV, de Muinck Keizer-Schrama SMPF, et al. Maternal thyroid autoimmunity during pregnancy and the risk of attention deficit/hyperactivity problems in children: the generation R study. Thyroid. 2012;22:178–86.
34. Chen L-M, Zhang Q, Si G-X, Chen Q-S, Ye E, Yu L-C, et al. Associations between thyroid autoantibody status and abnormal pregnancy outcomes in euthyroid women. Endocrine. 2015;48:924–8.
35. Monen L, Kuppens SM, Hasaart TH, Oosterbaan HP, Oei SG, Wijnen H, et al. Maternal thyrotropin is independently related to small for gestational age neonates at term. Clin Endocrinol. 2015;82:254–9.
36. Poppe K, Glinoer D, Van Steirteghem A, Tournaye H, Devroey P, Schiettecatte J, et al. Thyroid dysfunction and autoimmunity in infertile women. Thyroid. 2002;12:997–1001.
37. Ott J, Aust S, Kurz C, Nouri K, Wirth S, Huber JC, et al. Elevated antithyroid peroxidase antibodies indicating Hashimoto's thyroiditis are associated with the treatment response in infertile women with polycystic ovary syndrome. Fertil Steril. 2010;94:2895–7.

38. Wu H, Hong T, Gao H, Wang H. Effects of thyroid autoimmunity on pregnancy outcomes in euthyroid women receiving in vitro fertilization: a meta-analysis. Zhonghua Yi Xue Za Zhi. 2015;95:3770–4.
39. Toulis KA, Goulis DG, Venetis CA, Kolibianakis EM, Negro R, Tarlatzis BC, et al. Risk of spontaneous miscarriage in euthyroid women with thyroid autoimmunity undergoing IVF: a meta-analysis. Eur J Endocrinol. 2010;162:643–52.
40. Venables A, Wong W, Way M, Homer HA. Thyroid autoimmunity and IVF/ICSI outcomes in euthyroid women: a systematic review and meta-analysis. Reprod Biol Endocrinol. 2020;18:120.
41. Dhillon-Smith RK, Middleton LJ, Sunner KK, Cheed V, Baker K, Farrell-Carver S, et al. Levothyroxine in women with thyroid peroxidase antibodies before conception. N Engl J Med. 2019;380:1316–25.
42. Nazarpour S, Ramezani Tehrani F, Simbar M, Tohidi M, Alavi Majd H, Azizi F. Effects of levothyroxine treatment on pregnancy outcomes in pregnant women with autoimmune thyroid disease. Eur J Endocrinol. 2017;176:253–65.
43. Wang H, Gao H, Chi H, Zeng L, Xiao W, Wang Y, et al. Effect of levothyroxine on miscarriage among women with Normal thyroid function and thyroid autoimmunity undergoing in vitro fertilization and embryo transfer: a randomized clinical trial. JAMA. 2017;318:2190–8.
44. Casey BM, Thom EA, Peaceman AM, Varner MW, Sorokin Y, Hirtz DG, et al. Treatment of subclinical hypothyroidism or hypothyroxinemia in pregnancy. N Engl J Med. 2017;376:815–25.
45. Lazarus JH, Bestwick JP, Channon S, Paradice R, Maina A, Rees R, et al. Antenatal thyroid screening and childhood cognitive function. N Engl J Med. 2012;366:493–501.
46. Xie J, Jiang L, Sadhukhan A, Yang S, Yao Q, Zhou P, et al. Effect of antithyroid antibodies on women with recurrent miscarriage: a meta-analysis. Am J Reprod Immunol. 2020;83:e13238.
47. Contempre B, Dumont JE, Denef JF, Many MC. Effects of selenium deficiency on thyroid necrosis, fibrosis and proliferation: a possible role in myxoedematous cretinism. Eur J Endocrinol. 1995;133:99–109.
48. Gärtner R, Gasnier BCH, Dietrich JW, Krebs B, Angstwurm MWA. Selenium supplementation in patients with autoimmune thyroiditis decreases thyroid peroxidase antibodies concentrations. J Clin Endocrinol Metab. 2002;87:1687–91.
49. Fan Y, Xu S, Zhang H, Cao W, Wang K, Chen G, et al. Selenium supplementation for autoimmune thyroiditis: a systematic review and meta-analysis. Int J Endocrinol. 2014;2014:904573.
50. Karanikas G, Schuetz M, Kontur S, Duan H, Kommata S, Schoen R, et al. No immunological benefit of selenium in consecutive patients with autoimmune thyroiditis. Thyroid. 2008;18:7–12.
51. Negro R, Greco G, Mangieri T, Pezzarossa A, Dazzi D, Hassan H. The influence of selenium supplementation on postpartum thyroid status in pregnant women with thyroid peroxidase autoantibodies. J Clin Endocrinol Metab. 2007;92:1263–8.
52. Mao J, Pop VJ, Bath SC, Vader HL, Redman CWG, Rayman MP. Effect of low-dose selenium on thyroid autoimmunity and thyroid function in UK pregnant women with mild-to-moderate iodine deficiency. Eur J Nutr. 2016;55:55–61.
53. Stranges S, Marshall JR, Natarajan R, Donahue RP, Trevisan M, Combs GF, et al. Effects of long-term selenium supplementation on the incidence of type 2 diabetes: a randomized trial. Ann Intern Med. 2007;147:217–23.
54. Litwicka K, Arrivi C, Varricchio MT, Mencacci C, Greco E. In women with thyroid autoimmunity, does low-dose prednisolone administration, compared with no adjuvant therapy, improve in vitro fertilization clinical results? J Obstet Gynaecol Res. 2015;41:722–8.
55. Turi A, Giannubilo SR, Zanconi S, Mascetti A, Tranquilli AL. Preconception steroid treatment in infertile women with antithyroid autoimmunity undergoing ovarian stimulation and intrauterine insemination: a double-blind, randomized, prospective cohort study. Clin Ther. 2010;32:2415–21.
56. Stricker RB, Steinleitner A, Bookoff CN, Weckstein LN, Winger EE. Successful treatment of immunologic abortion with low-dose intravenous immunoglobulin. Fertil Steril. 2000;73:536–40.

57. Kiprov DD, Nachtigall RD, Weaver RC, Jacobson A, Main EK, Garovoy MR. The use of intravenous immunoglobulin in recurrent pregnancy loss associated with combined alloimmune and autoimmune abnormalities. Am J Reprod Immunol. 1996;36:228–34.
58. Vaquero E, Lazzarin N, De Carolis C, Valensise H, Moretti C, Ramanini C. Mild thyroid abnormalities and recurrent spontaneous abortion: diagnostic and therapeutical approach. Am J Reprod Immunol. 2000;43:204–8.

Hypothyroidism in Pregnancy

5

Ritesh Kumar, Ayan Roy, and Vahid S. Bharmal

5.1 Introduction

Hypothyroidism is one of the most common endocrine disorders that complicate pregnancy. Overt hypothyroidism (OH) is responsible for the majority of the cases. But the incidence of subclinical hypothyroidism (SCH) is increasing significantly due to the increased availability of tests and increased awareness among clinicians resulting in more screening at the onset of pregnancy. The combined prevalence of hypothyroidism (both OH and SCH) may reach up to 4–7% in a specific population (Western). The impact of OH is understandably more significant with respect to foeto-maternal outcomes, whereas the effect of SCH is less well defined. Hypothyroidism in pregnancy may be identified as a result of routine screening or when an already-known patient of hypothyroidism conceives. It is important to note that majority of the guidelines do not recommend routine screening of TSH in the first trimester of pregnancy; rather at-risk screening may be more suitable in low- and middle-income countries. Still, in clinical practice,

Authors' Contributions: RK and VB have drafted the overt hypothyroidism in pregnancy, and AR has drafted the subclinical hypothyroidism part, respectively. All the authors have edited and approved the final manuscript.

R. Kumar
Endocrinology, Institute of Medical Sciences, Banaras Hindu University, Varanasi, Uttar Pradesh, India

A. Roy (✉)
Endocrinology and Metabolism, All India Institute of Medical Sciences, Kalyani, West Bengal, India

V. S. Bharmal
Bhailal Amin General Hospital, Gorwa, Vadodara, India

H. Sagili et al. (eds.), *Thyroid Disease in Pregnancy - A Guide to Clinical Management*, https://doi.org/10.1007/978-981-99-5423-0_5

screening of TSH is widely used during pregnancy. An increasing maternal childbearing age may also contribute to the generalised increase in the prevalence of elevated TSH during pregnancy.

Hitherto, the SCH definition is heterogeneous and relies on the upper limit of the normal cutoff of a population-specific TSH, and the definition is problematic as various ranges have been used. This situation is more complicated in places where there are no trimester and population-specific cutoffs available to use. Widely used international guidelines like the American thyroid association (ATA) suggest a normal upper limit of 4 mIU/ml for TSH. SCH treatment is based on the individualisation of levothyroxine (LT4) therapy based on certain associated patient-specific factors. As we discuss further, there are many existing knowledge gaps in the management of SCH and the impact of normalisation of TSH on the foeto-maternal outcome, which is considered as the treatment goal of SCH. Nevertheless, a thorough knowledge of OH and SCH definitions, consequences, and management is required, and we discuss those pertinent issues in this chapter. We also provide simplified algorithms for managing this common endocrinopathy encountered during pregnancy.

5.2 Overt Hypothyroidism in Pregnancy

5.2.1 Definition and Epidemiology

OH is characterised by an elevated TSH with low free thyroxine (fT4) concentration [1]. The exact cutoff point of TSH above which OH is diagnosed in the presence of normal fT4 remains less defined, but a TSH cutoff of more than 10 mIU/ml suggests OH (ATA 2017).

OH affects approximately 1–2% of women in the reproductive age group [2]. Most pregnant women are on treatment before conception. OH diagnosed during pregnancy is unusual but can be present in 0.3–0.5% of screened women. The prevalence is often higher in moderately iodine-deficient regions and can be as high as 4.58% [3]. Apart from iodine deficiency, other factors behind the development of OH are autoimmunity, obesity, and ethnicity, namely White Caucasians [4–6]. The various etiology of OH during pregnancy in decreasing frequency include (1) autoimmune thyroiditis (Hashimoto's thyroiditis), (2) post-radioactive iodine ablation in thyrotoxicosis (Graves' disease or toxic multinodular goitre or toxic adenoma), (3) post-surgical hypothyroidism, (4) iodine deficiency, and rarely (5) central hypothyroidism and (6) congenital hypothyroidism. Thus, such patients require proper preconceptional care including thorough history of thyroid surgery or radioiodine ablation treatment.

5.2.2 Maternal Adverse Outcomes of Overt Hypothyroidism during Pregnancy

Studies are limited to the effects of OH on pregnancy outcomes. Observational studies have shown an increased risk of miscarriage in untreated or inadequately treated OH [7, 8]. The chance of miscarriage was four times higher in women with TSH greater than 10 mIU/L than those with TSH 1–2.5 mIU/L [9]. Similarly, an abortion rate of 4% in euthyroid versus 31.4% in hypothyroid women ($p < 0.0001$) was also observed [7]. Elevated TSH in the second and third trimesters was found to be associated with increased foetal death (odds ratio (OR) 4.4, 95% confidence interval (CI) 1.9–9.5) [10].

A study compared the rate of abortion and premature delivery in 103 severe hypothyroid (defined by TSH > 20 mIU/ml) pregnant women with 205 euthyroid pregnant women [11]. In this study, the maximum serum TSH was 150, and the mean duration of hypothyroidism during pregnancy was 21.2 ± 13.2 weeks. All patients were treated with LT4 during pregnancy, but TSH levels during pregnancy were elevated in 34.9% of cases. The reported rates of abortions were 7.8%, premature deliveries in 2.9% in hypothyroid pregnant women, while euthyroid pregnant women had an abortion in 9.3%, and premature delivery in 1.5% without any significant differences. Similarly, Montoro et al. found a single case of foetal death at 29 weeks of pregnancy out of 11 severe hypothyroid pregnant women (mean TSH was 105). This suggests that even women with severe hypothyroidism may conceive and sustain pregnancy successfully [12].

Furthermore, elevated TSH in the late first trimester was associated with late-onset preeclampsia after 34 weeks of gestation [13]. In a small group of pregnant women with OH, maternal complications were commonly seen, namely anaemia (31%), preeclampsia (44%), placental abruption (19%), postpartum haemorrhage (19%), and cardiac dysfunction [14, 15]. The observed gestational hypertension seen in OH can be due to an increase in the peripheral resistance and arterial wall thickness related to OH. Endothelial dysfunction also is a notable contributor. Importantly, these pathological changes of OH during pregnancy are often reversed by the treatment with LT4.

In summary, OH has a definite association with various adverse maternal outcomes like preeclampsia, gestational hypertension, anaemia, placental anomalies, and postpartum haemorrhage (Table 5.1).

Table 5.1 Effect of hypothyroidism on maternal and foetal outcomes

Maternal outcome	Foetal outcome
Spontaneous abortion [8, 10, 13, 14]	Low birth weight [14, 15]
Preeclampsia, eclampsia, gestational hypertension [13–15]	Low intelligence quotient, neuropsychological, and cognitive impairment [16, 17]
Placental abruption [14]	Small hippocampal volume and decreased memory [18]
Preterm delivery [14, 15]	Death
Postpartum haemorrhage [14]	

These complications are directly related to three principal factors: (1) the degree of hypothyroidism, the higher the TSH it is more likely that adverse outcome can be poor; (2) the duration of the OH before the initiation of therapy, a longer duration can impact pregnancy more adversely; and finally (3) the treatment status and regular follow up of the patient.

5.2.3 Foetal Outcomes of Overt Hypothyroidism in Pregnancy

The foetal thyroid gland starts producing thyroid hormone from 16 to 20 weeks of gestation. Thyroid hormones are required for the optimal development of multiple organ systems, including the brain. During the first trimester, thyroid hormone supply is dependent mainly on the transplacental passage of maternal T4 [19]. So, maternal OH is associated with an increased risk of preterm delivery, including very preterm delivery (before 32 weeks), low birth weight, neuropsychological and cognitive impairment in the child [7, 14–17]. Premature delivery and low birth weight were reported in 20–31% of cases of hypothyroidism during pregnancy. But these results were confounded by gestational hypertension, preeclampsia, and eclampsia which were also prevalent in hypothyroid mothers [7, 14].

Thyroid hormones are necessary for neuronal cell differentiation and migration, myelin formation, and synaptogenesis [20]. Thyroid hormone deficiency may lead to neurological impairment, especially during the first trimester. Haddow et al. assessed the developmental problem in children aged 7–9 years whose mothers had hypothyroidism during pregnancy [17]. Out of 62, 48 were not treated during the pregnancy. The total intelligence quotient (IQ) score of their children was 7 points lower than those of 124 match control children, and 19% of them had a score of less than 85 compared to 5% of control. Similarly, significantly smaller hippocampal volume and decreased memory in the offspring of hypothyroid mothers were also observed [18]. Hippocampal volumes negatively correlated with maternal third-trimester TSH levels and positively correlated with maternal T4.

5.2.4 Management of Overt Hypothyroidism in Pregnancy

ATA recommends the management of OH as soon as possible with the goal of normalisation of TSH. Observational studies have shown that the earlier the achievement of euthyroidism, the lower the pregnancy complication rate. The best evidence for treatment is derived from a large observational study that included 20,000 pregnant women [21]. This study demonstrated that treatment of OH resulted in the normalisation of the risk of adverse maternal and neonatal outcomes.

The management of OH during pregnancy can be subdivided into the following three strata:

1. OH with adequate treatment preconceptionally (TSH in the cutoff range while entering pregnancy).

2. OH but inadequately treated preconceptionally (TSH above upper normal limit (UNL) entering into pregnancy).
3. Newly diagnosed OH during pregnancy (as a result of screening).

5.2.4.1 Women with Pre-existing Hypothyroidism with Adequate Treatment Preconceptionally

Women with pre-existing hypothyroidism who have normal TSH during the preconception period often require an increase in the LT4 replacement dose, particularly in the first trimester of the pregnancy. However, the dose increment may be related to the level of TSH also, as it was seen that, among pregnant women with preconception TSH less than 1.2 mIU/l, only 17% required a dose increase in LT4 (LT4), while 50% with preconception TSH of 1.2–2.5 mIU/l required a dose increase [1]. One trial (THERAPY) showed that doubling the pre-pregnancy dose of LT4 on 2 days a week (29% total increase) successfully prevented maternal hypothyroidism in 85% of women in the first trimester with very minimal risk of TSH suppression. Based on this data, an empirical dose increase of 30–50% is recommended over and above the ongoing dose of LT4 as soon as pregnancy is confirmed in a hypothyroid woman. A 4 weekly monitoring of TSH is sufficient to maintain euthyroidism in the first 20 weeks of pregnancy (Fig. 5.1) [22]. For women with no residual thyroid function or athyreosis (following thyroidectomy and radioactive ablation), the total increase in LT4 dose may be higher (45% approximately) [22]. After 20 weeks of gestation, thyroxine-binding globulin and HCG (human chorionic gonadotropin) concentrations stabilise. Therefore, LT4 requirement usually plateaus after 20 weeks of gestation. But other factors like iron deficiency and iron supplementation also require an increased LT4 dose [23]. Therefore, thyroid function should be repeated at least two times after mid-gestation at 28 and 34 weeks. Once the TSH level stabilises between 0. and 2.5 mU/l, the final LT4 dosage requirement may be different in

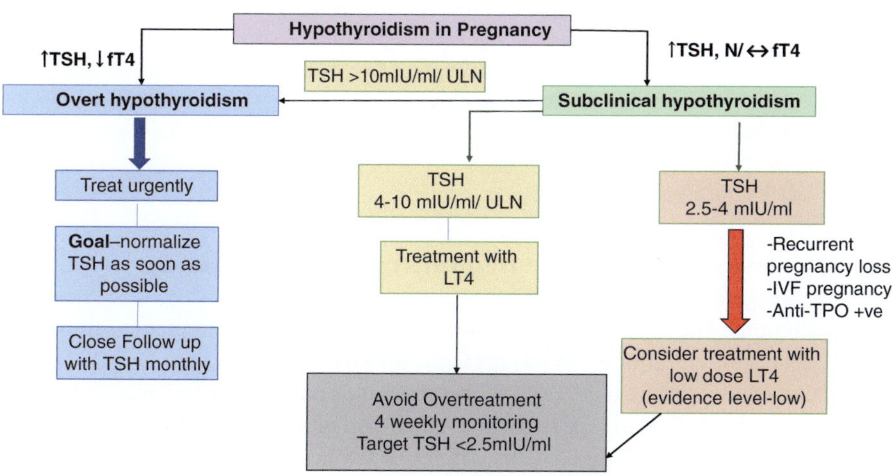

Fig. 5.1 Simplified approach to hypothyroidism management in pregnancy

the clinical context of the mother, e.g., higher dose in post-ablative hypothyroidism [24].

Case Scenario 1

A 27-year-old lady, a known case of primary hypothyroidism is on LT4 75 mcg/day. Her latest TSH is 3.5 mIU/ml. She now wants to conceive. What is the next best step in her management?

Answer: Continue LT4 75 mcg. As soon as the pregnancy is confirmed, a dose increment to 88–100 mcg is advisable (an increment of 25–30% of preconceptional dose). This should be followed up with monthly TSH with a <2.5-mIU/ml target.

5.2.4.2 Women with Pre-existing Hypothyroidism with Inadequate Treatment Preconceptionally and in Early Pregnancy

There are two management approaches in such cases, but robust evidence is lacking. Firstly, an increase in the LT4 dose by a greater magnitude has a risk of transient mild hyperthyroidism, then the dose needs to be titrated to a maintenance level. The second approach is to increase the dose gradually with frequent monitoring of TSH. However, treating women with a higher LT4 dose carries the risk of overshooting FT4, and there have been few associations of higher FT4 with autistic spectrum disorder [25, 26].

Case Scenario 2

A 32-year-old patient, Mrs. S is on 75 mcg LT4 supplementation. She had a history of radioiodine ablation of the thyroid due to Graves' disease 4 years back. Her current TSH is 8.9 mIU/ml, and she reported a positive urinary pregnancy test. What is the next best step for management?

Answer: This lady has post-ablative hypothyroidism and has inadequately controlled TSH while entering into pregnancy. Her dose of LT4 should be increased to 100 mcg/day with TSH following up four weekly. The aim is to normalise TSH as soon as possible.

5.2.4.3 Management of Overt Hypothyroidism That Is Newly Diagnosed in Pregnancy

This is a unique situation and often requires careful attention. A higher starting dose of LT4 dose is often required in this scenario for OH. A dose as high as 2.0–2.4 ug/kg, instead of the routine dose used in the general population (1.6–1.8 ug/kg), usually is recommended. Retrospective analysis of patients with OH during pregnancy has shown that with an initial LT4 dose of 2.33 ± 0.59 ug/kg/day, 76.92% of patients reached the TSH target within 5.3 ± 1.8 weeks. In addition, no significant difference between the initial and final dose was observed [27]. Increased surveillance for maternal hypertension, preeclampsia, and foetal growth restriction is recommended for OH women diagnosed during the first trimester. After delivery, most women require the pre-pregnancy dose of LT4. However, some women following delivery may need a higher LT4 dose than pre-pregnancy because of postpartum progression of autoimmune thyroiditis [28].

Case Scenario 3

A 34-year-old lady was found to have TSH of 52 mIU/ml on routine screening during 12 weeks of pregnancy. Her mother also has primary hypothyroidism. What is the next best step in management?

Answer: Continuation of pregnancy with immediate start of LT4 (2–2.4 mcg/kg/day). Rapid achievement of euthyroidism with monthly monitoring of TSH and foetal monitoring as per the recommendations.

5.2.5 The Issue of Medical Termination of Pregnancy in Overt Hypothyroidism

If OH is diagnosed before 20 weeks of gestation and adequately treated with proper monitoring, the risk of maternal and foetal complications is significantly reduced. So, all patients ideally should be treated with LT4 as per guidelines. If overt hypothyroidism is severe, medical termination of pregnancy can be considered if there is a request from the patient considering various factors. Several factors influence medical termination of pregnancy in OH like the severity of hypothyroidism, past history of infertility, miscarriage/foetal loss, congenital malformation, offspring with intellectual impairment, and family history of congenital malformation and intellectual impairment [29].

5.3 Subclinical Hypothyroidism in Pregnancy

5.3.1 Definition and Epidemiology

There has been no such debated topic as SCH, including its cause and consequences and treatment goals and outcomes. SCH is defined as the elevation of serum TSH from the ULN while serum FT4 is still normal [30]. Whereas the opposite state of normal TSH and decreased FT4 levels during pregnancy are denoted as isolated maternal hypothyroxinaemia (IH). This definition is often variable across studies as the cutoff of the ULN differs based on population or assay platform use. The ATA 2017 guideline [31] suggests a population and trimester-specific cutoff for pregnancy to be used. However, in many countries, population-specific cutoffs are not available. In that scenario, a cutoff using similar to but from other populations can be taken, or a TSH value of 4.0 mIU/L can be used as an upper reference range. However, earlier studies have estimated SCH prevalence using a TSH value of 2.5 mIU/L as the ULN also. Till a consensus is reached, the ULN of 4.0 mIU/L in the absence of normal reference data can serve as a reference for SCH.

The prevalence of SCH depends on several factors like ethnicity, body mass index, age of the population, the assay platform used to measure TSH, iodine status of the population, and finally, the cutoff chosen to define the ULN. Approximately the prevalence ranges from 2 to 15% in different studies, including different populations, and is a heterogeneous finding mostly driven by the use of different assays across studies. Understandably, the prevalence increases when universal screening for TSH is adopted, and the cutoff is lowered to 2.5 mIU/L.

5.3.2 Consequences of SCH in Pregnancy

The major impact of SCH remains on the obstetric outcomes as compared to IH, where offspring's outcomes are more often affected. This finding is in stark contrast with OH, which is associated with significant morbidity in both mothers and neonates. However, the evidence of SCH on pregnancy outcomes is based on small observational studies implying low-quality evidence. A recent study analysing over 8000 pregnancies and their offspring showed that a maternal TSH level of more than 4 mIU/L was associated with twofold increased risk of prematurity [risk ratio (RR) 2.17,(95% CI 1.15–4.07)] and neonatal respiratory distress syndrome [RR 2.83 (95% CI 1.02–7.86)] when compared to TSH levels ≤4 mIU/L [32]. Moreover, foetal loss, preeclampsia/eclampsia, and low birth weight babies were more in the former group (TSH > 4 mIU/L), but preterm delivery, gestational hypertension or diabetes, abruptio placentae, caesarean section, or neonatal intensive care unit admissions was similar to TSH < 4 mIU/L. Earlier prospective studies also have reported increased miscarriage rates even in the range of TSH of 2.5–5.0 mIU/L [33]. However, these results were negated by other studies [34]. A recent large meta-analysis showed a higher preterm birth in the SCH cohort compared to a normal cohort [OR, 1.29 [95% CI, 1.01–1.64 [35], especially in thyroid peroxidase antibody (TPO Ab)-positive women. However, maternal SCH status was found to have no impact on offspring's IQ and brain development [36]. Thus, in summary, SCH may have an impact on pregnancy loss and preterm birth, but this is often based on conflicting evidence and no universal TSH cutoff has been accepted in this context.

Whether SCH adversely affects the outcome of assisted reproductive technology pregnancies is an important consideration. The outcome may not differ between LT4 treated versus nontreated patients at the TSH range of 2.5–4.5 mIU/L. However, when TSH elevation is in the range of more than 4.5–5 mIU/L, LT4 treatment has shown a beneficial impact in terms of improved clinical pregnancy rate, decrease in the miscarriage rate, and improved delivery rate.

5.3.3 Pathophysiology of SCH

The principal question remains whether SCH can result in adverse foeto-maternal outcomes. The postulations revolve around autoimmunity as the pivot and whether SCH is a maladaptive state of the thyroid axis in pregnancy is not fully elucidated.

In normal pregnancy, TSH levels are suppressed in the first trimester due to the rising titre of HCG secreted from the placenta. However, interestingly, the normal linear relation of TSH and fT4 in response to peak hCG appears to be blunted in TPO-positive women with higher preterm birth and thus pointing to the role of autoimmunity in adverse pregnancy outcomes [37]. On the other hand, if it is believed that if SCH is a result of the failure of the maternal thyroid tissue to raise thyroid hormone levels adequately in the face of extra demand of pregnancy, treatment of SCH aimed to normalise TSH levels should have shown to reduce the adverse outcome. However, this is not supported by consistent evidence, including a few recent randomised controlled trials. Moreover, a combination of TPO Ab positivity and SCH may have a more unfavourable metabolic effect on the pregnancy outcome. Sometimes, SCH may reflect more generalised autoimmunity in a patient similar to systemic lupus erythematosus or autoimmune polyglandular syndrome, including type 1 diabetes [38]. The recent discovery of the TPO antigen in the ovarian follicle might point towards a direct role of this antigen in the pregnancy outcome in future studies.

5.3.4 Management of SCH in Pregnancy

The management of SCH in pregnancy is individualised and based on moderate evidence. The TSH level at which treatment should be started is debated. Whenever available, a population-specific ULN is useful. However, if unavailable, a TSH threshold of 4–4.5 mIU/L can be used as a surrogate. The ATA guideline suggests a treatment threshold of 4 mIU/L [39]. At the TSH level of 2.5 to UNL of 4 mIU/L, antibody status and other significant parameters are important in decision-making. In the presence of TPOAb positivity, recurrent pregnancy loss, or IVF pregnancy, treatment of SCH with LT4 is considered [30] (Fig. 5.1).

However, the beneficial impact of treatment on pregnancy outcomes should be weighed against the adverse outcome of the foetus in case of increased FT4 due to overtreatment. Importantly two recently published trials (TABLET and T4LIFE) failed to show any beneficial impact of LT4 treatment on the live birth outcome in anti-TPO Ab-positive women with normal TSH [40, 41]. A low dose therapy with 25–50 mcg of LT4 should be used in such circumstances, and monitoring of TSH and FT4 to be done every month. Importantly, an adequate daily iodine intake of 250 mcg should be maintained. In TPOAb-negative women, treatment with LT4 did not reduce pregnancy complications at the TSH range of 2.5–4.0 mIU/L, whereas benefit was demonstrated in treating TSH more than 4 mIU/L [42].

Case Scenario 4a

A 26-year-old lady came with TSH of 5.9 mIU/ml in the first trimester of pregnancy. She had a history of missed abortions at 8 weeks. Her anti-TPO antibody is strongly positive. How should she be approached?

Answer: Start LT4 25–50 mcg per day and monitor TSH monthly with a target TSH of less than 4 mIU/ml.

Case Scenario 4b

A 26-year-old lady came with TSH of 3.3 mIU/ml in the first trimester of pregnancy. She had a history of missed abortions at 8 weeks. Her anti-TPO antibody is strongly positive. How should she be approached?

Answer: The latest randomised controlled trials showed no benefit of LT4 supplementations in such a scenario. So, watchful observation with serial monitoring of TSH can be employed.

Key Messages

- OH has adverse effects on maternal and foetal outcomes if left untreated or inadequately treated.
- The ultimate goal of management of OH in pregnancy is a rapid achievement of euthyroidism and maintenance of euthyroidism during preconception and throughout pregnancy.
- On the other hand, SCH remains an important issue. Definition of SCH requires a population-specific cutoff.
- The treatment effects in the lowest TSH range are not substantiated by the evidence, but treatment reduces maternal complications when a higher TSH cutoff is used for the treatment initiation.
- Treating TPOAb-positive women with normal TSH and LT4 is debated and requirs individualisation.

Conflict of interest Nil.

Funding
Nil.

References

1. Abalovich M, Alcaraz G, Kleiman-Rubinsztein J, Pavlove MM, Cornelio C, Levalle O, et al. The relationship of preconception thyrotropin levels to requirements for increasing the LT4 dose during pregnancy in women with primary hypothyroidism. Thyroid. 2010;20(10):1175–8.
2. Bryant SN, Nelson DB, McIntire DD, Casey BM, Cunningham FG. An analysis of population-based prenatal screening for overt hypothyroidism. Am J Obstet Gynecol. 2015;213(4):565e1–6.
3. Sahu MT, Das V, Mittal S, Agarwal A, Sahu M. Overt and subclinical thyroid dysfunction among Indian pregnant women and its effect on maternal and fetal outcome. Arch Gynecol Obstet. 2010;281(2):215–20.
4. Han C, Li C, Mao J, Wang W, Xie X, Zhou W, et al. High body mass index is an indicator of maternal hypothyroidism, hypothyroxinemia, and thyroid-peroxidase antibody positivity during early pregnancy. Biomed Res Int. 2015;2015:351831.

5. Olmos RD, Figueiredo RC, Aquino EM, Lotufo PA, Bensenor IM. Gender, race and socioeconomic influence on diagnosis and treatment of thyroid disorders in the Brazilian longitudinal study of adult health (ELSA-Brasil). Brazilian journal of medical and biological research =. Revista brasileira de pesquisas medicas e biologicas. 2015;48(8):751–8.
6. Hollowell JG, Staehling NW, Flanders WD, Hannon WH, Gunter EW, Spencer CA, et al. Serum TSH, T (4), and thyroid antibodies in the United States population (1988 to 1994): National Health and NutritionExamination survey (NHANES III). J Clin Endocrinol Metab. 2002;87(2):489–99.
7. Abalovich M, Gutierrez S, Alcaraz G, et al. Overt and subclinical hypothyroidism complicating pregnancy. Thyroid. 2002;12:63.
8. Hallengren B, Lantz M, Andreasson B, Grennert L. Pregnant women on thyroxine substitution are often dysregulated in early pregnancy. Thyroid. 2009;19:391.
9. Taylor PN, Minassian C, Rehman A, Iqbal A, Draman MS, Hamilton W, et al. TSH levels and risk of miscarriage in women on long-term levothyroxine: a community-based study. J Clin Endocrinol Metabol. 2014;99:3895–902.
10. Allan WC, Haddow JE, Palomaki GE, Williams JR, Mitchell ML, Hermos RJ, et al. Maternal thyroid deficiency and pregnancy complications: implications for population screening. J Med Screen. 2000;7:127–30.
11. Hirsch D, Levy S, Nadler V, Kopel V, Shainberg B, Toledano Y. Pregnancy outcomes in women with severe hypothyroidism. Eur J Endocrinol. 2013;169:313–20.
12. Montoro M, Collea JV, Frasier SD, Mestman JH. Successful outcome of pregnancy in women with hypothyroidism. Ann Intern Med. 1981;94(1):31–4.
13. Ashoor G, Maiz N, Rotas M, Kametas NA, Nicolaides KH. Maternal thyroid function at 11 to 13 weeks of gestation and subsequent development of preeclampsia. Prenat Diagn. 2010;30(11):1032–8.
14. Davis LE, Leveno KJ, Cunningham FG. Hypothyroidism complicating pregnancy. Obstet Gynecol. 1988;72(1):108–12.
15. Leung AS, Millar LK, Koonings PP, Montoro M, Mestman JH. Perinatal outcome in hypothyroid pregnancies. Obstet Gynecol. 1993;81:349–53.
16. LaFranchi SH, Haddow JE, Hollowell JG. Is thyroid inadequacy during gestation a risk factor for adverse pregnancy and developmental outcomes? Thyroid. 2005;15(1):60–71.
17. Haddow JE, Palomaki GE, Allan WC, Williams JR, Knight GJ, Gagnon J, et al. Maternal thyroid deficiency during pregnancy and subsequent neuropsychological development of the child. N Engl J Med. 1999;341(8):549–55.
18. Willoughby KA, McAndrews MP, Rovet JF. Effects of maternal hypothyroidism on offspring hippocampus and memory. Thyroid. 2014;24:576.
19. Thorpe-Beeston JG, Nicolaides KH, Felton CV, Butler J, McGregor AM. Maturation of the secretion of thyroid hormone and thyroid stimulating hormone in the fetus. The New England Journal of Medicine. 1991;324(8):532–6.
20. Bernal J. Thyroid hormone receptors in brain development and function. Nat Clin Pract Endocrinol Metab. 2007;3:249–59.
21. Idris I, Srinivasan R, Simm A, Page RC. Maternal hypothyroidism in early and late gestation: effects on neonatal and obstetric outcome. Clin Endocrinol. 2005;63(5):560–5.
22. Assa L, Marqusee E, Fawcett R, Alexander EK. Thyroid hormone early adjustment in pregnancy (the THERAPY) trial. J Clin Endocrinol Metab. 2010;95(7):3234–41.
23. Li S, Gao X, Wei Y, Zhu G, Yang C. The relationship between iron deficiency and thyroid function in Chinese women during early pregnancy. J Nutr Sci Vitaminol. 2016;62(6):397–401.
24. Verga U, Bergamaschi S, Cortelazzi D, Ronzoni S, Marconi AM, Beck-Peccoz P. Adjustment of L-T4 substitutive therapy in pregnant women with subclinical, overt or post-ablative hypothyroidism. Clin Endocrinol. 2009;70:798–802.
25. Andersen SL, Laurberg P, Wu CS, Olsen J. Attention deficit hyperactivity disorder and autism spectrum disorder in children born to mothers with thyroid dysfunction: a Danish nationwide cohort study. BJOG. 2014;121(11):1365–74.

26. Levie D, Korevaar TIM, Bath SC, Dalmau-Bueno A, Murcia M, Espada M, et al. Thyroid function in early pregnancy, child IQ, and autistic traits: a meta-analysis of individual participant data. J Clin Endocrinol Metab. 2018;103(8):2967–79.
27. Abalovich M, Vázquez A, Alcaraz G, Kitaigrodsky A, Szuman G, Calabrese C, Astarita G, Frydman M, Gutiérrez S. Adequate levothyroxine doses for the treatment of hypothyroidism newly discovered during pregnancy. Thyroid. 2013 Nov;23(11):1479–83.
28. Galofré JC, Haber RS, Mitchell AA, Pessah R, Davies TF. Increased postpartum thyroxine replacement in Hashimoto's thyroiditis. Thyroid. 2010;20:901–8.
29. Kalra S, Ganie MA, Unnikrishnan AG. Overt hypothyroidism in pregnancy: can we consider medical termination of pregnancy? Ind J Endocrinol Metab. 2013 Mar;17(2):197–9.
30. Taylor PN, Muller I, Nana M, Velasco I, Lazarus JH. Indications for treatment of subclinical hypothyroidism and isolated hypothyroxinaemia in pregnancy. Best Pract Res Clin Endocrinol Metab. 2020;34(4):101436.
31. Alexander EK, Pearce EN, Brent GA, et al. Guidelines of the American Thyroid Association for the diagnosis and Management of Thyroid Disease during Pregnancy and the postpartum [published correction appears in thyroid. 2017 Sep;27(9):1212]. Thyroid. 2017;27(3):315–89.
32. Lee SY, Cabral HJ, Aschengrau A, Pearce EN. Associations between maternal thyroid function in pregnancy and obstetric and perinatal outcomes. J Clin Endocrinol Metab. 2020 May 1;105(5):e2015–23.
33. Negro R, Schwartz A, Gismondi R, Tinelli A, Mangieri T, Stagnaro-Green A. Increased pregnancy loss rate in thyroid antibody negative women with TSH levels between 2.5 and 5.0 in the first trimester of pregnancy. J Clin Endocrinol Metab. 2010 Sep;95(9):E44–8.
34. Cleary-Goldman J, Malone FD, Lambert-Messerlian G, Sullivan L, Canick J, MD for the FASTER Consortium, et al. Maternal Thyroid Hypofunction and Pregnancy Outcome. Obstet Gynecol. 2008;112(1):85–92.
35. Consortium on Thyroid and Pregnancy—Study Group on Preterm Birth, TIM K, Derakhshan A, Taylor PN, Meima M, Chen L, Bliddal S, Carty DM, et al. Association of Thyroid Function Test Abnormalities and Thyroid Autoimmunity with preterm birth: a systematic review and meta-analysis. JAMA. 2019 Aug 20;322(7):632–41.
36. Korevaar TI, Muetzel R, Medici M, Chaker L, Jaddoe VW, de Rijke YB, et al. Association of maternal thyroid function during early pregnancy with offspring IQ and brain morphology in childhood: a population-based prospective cohort study. Lancet Diabetes Endocrinol. 2016 Jan;4(1):35–43.
37. Tim I, Korevaar M, Steegers EAP, Pop VJ, Maarten A, et al. Thyroid autoimmunity impairs the thyroidal response to human chorionic gonadotropin: two population-based prospective cohort studies. J Clin Endocrinol Metab. 2017;102(1):69–77.
38. Brabant G, Peeters RP, Chan SY, Bernal J, Bouchard P, Salvatore D, et al. Management of subclinical hypothyroidism in pregnancy: are we too simplistic? Eur J Endocrinol. 2015;173:P1–11.
39. Alexander EK, Pearce EN, Brent GA, Brown RS, Chen H, Dosiou C, et al. 2017 guidelines of the American Thyroid Association for the diagnosis and Management of Thyroid Disease during Pregnancy and the postpartum. Thyroid. 2017;27:315–89.
40. van Dijk MM, Vissenberg R, Fliers E, van der Post JAM, van der Hoorn MP, et al. LT4 in euthyroid thyroid peroxidase antibody positive women with recurrent pregnancy loss (T4LIFE trial): a multicentre, randomised, double-blind, placebo-controlled, phase 3 trial. Lancet Diabetes Endocrinol. 2022 Mar 14;S2213-8587(22):00045–6.
41. Dhillon-Smith RK, Middleton LJ, Sunner KK, Cheed V, Baker K, Farrell-Carver S, et al. LT4 in women with thyroid peroxidase antibodies before conception. N Engl J Med. 2019 Apr 4;380(14):1316–25.
42. Nazarpour S, Ramezani Tehrani F, Simbar M, Tohidi M, Minooee S, Rahmati M, Azizi F. Effects of LT4 on pregnant women with subclinical hypothyroidism, negative for thyroid peroxidase antibodies. J Clin Endocrinol Metab. 2018 Mar 1;103(3):926–35.

6 Hyperthyroidism and Pregnancy

Kripa Elizabeth Cherian and Vijaya Bhaskar Reddy Sagili

6.1 Introduction

Hyperthyroidism refers to excess thyroid hormones in the blood due to excess production of thyroid hormones by the thyroid gland. Hyperthyroidism in pregnancy should be diagnosed carefully in view of changes in thyroid function tests due to pregnancy itself. The symptoms of hyperthyroidism might mimic normal physiological changes in pregnancy and thus could pose a challenge to diagnosis. Moderate to severe hyperthyroidism can adversely affect pregnancy and the foetus. The diagnosis of hyperthyroidism in pregnancy requires careful attention to patient symptomatology, clinical features and laboratory tests. Early recognition and appropriate treatment of hyperthyroidism are crucial to ensure adequate maternal and foetal well-being during pregnancy [1].

Authors' Contributions: VBR and KEC have drafted the book chapter. Both authors have edited and approved the final manuscript.

K. E. Cherian
Department of Endocrinology, Christian Medical College and Hospital, Vellore, India

V. B. R. Sagili (✉)
Vijay Diabetes, Thyroid and Endocrine Clinic, Puducherry, India

H. Sagili et al. (eds.), *Thyroid Disease in Pregnancy - A Guide to Clinical Management*, https://doi.org/10.1007/978-981-99-5423-0_6

6.2 Physiology of Maternal and Foetal Thyroid in Pregnancy Relevant to Hyperthyroidism

As soon as pregnancy is established, the levels of human chorionic glycoprotein (hCG), a 37-kDa glycoprotein secreted by the syncytiotrophoblasts of the placenta increases and peaks by 8–11 weeks of gestation [2]. Bearing structural homology to thyroid stimulating hormone (TSH), it stimulates maternal TSH receptors on the thyroid gland leading to an increase in total thyroxine concentration, a transient increase in free thyroxine levels and suppression of TSH [3].

Physiologically, pregnancy witnesses an increase in thyroid binding globulin (TBG), a 54-KDa glycoprotein synthesised by the liver [4]. Under the influence of maternal oestrogen, TBG concentration increases a few weeks after conception and plateaus by mid-gestation. The mechanism of this increase is attributed to the increased rate of synthesis by the liver and decreased clearance of the protein from the plasma [5]. The increase in TBG leads to higher binding of total thyroxine, a mild decrease in the concentration of free thyroxine and a consequent rise in TSH, which is apparent by the second trimester of pregnancy [6].

The deiodinases expressed by the placenta also play a role in the thyroid economy of pregnancy. In early pregnancy, placental deiodinase 2 ensures increased conversion of tetra-iodothyronine (T4) to tri-iodothyronine (T3) and this is responsible for maintaining adequate intra-placental T3 for trophoblast development and differentiation. Placental deiodinase 3 on the other hand increases conversion of T4 to rT3 (reverse T3) and T3 to di-iodothyronine (T2). As this prevents activation of T4 and inactivates T3, the foetus is protected from excess maternal thyroid hormones, while there is an increased maternal hormone demand [7].

During pregnancy, there is a reduction in the maternal iodide pool related to increased production of thyroid hormones, increased renal clearance and increased transfer to the developing foetus. Thus, the various physiological changes that occur during pregnancy are meant to ensure an optimal pregnancy outcome and promote normal development of the offspring [7]. The changes in the thyroid axis in normal pregnancy are summarised in Fig. 6.1.

Thyrotoxicosis refers to excess thyroid hormones in the blood either due to excess production (hyperthyroidism) or excess release from destruction of thyroid follicles (thyroiditis) or exogenous thyroid hormones (overtreatment or factitious). Hyperthyroidism has to be differentiated from thyrotoxicosis due to other causes, where production is not increased.

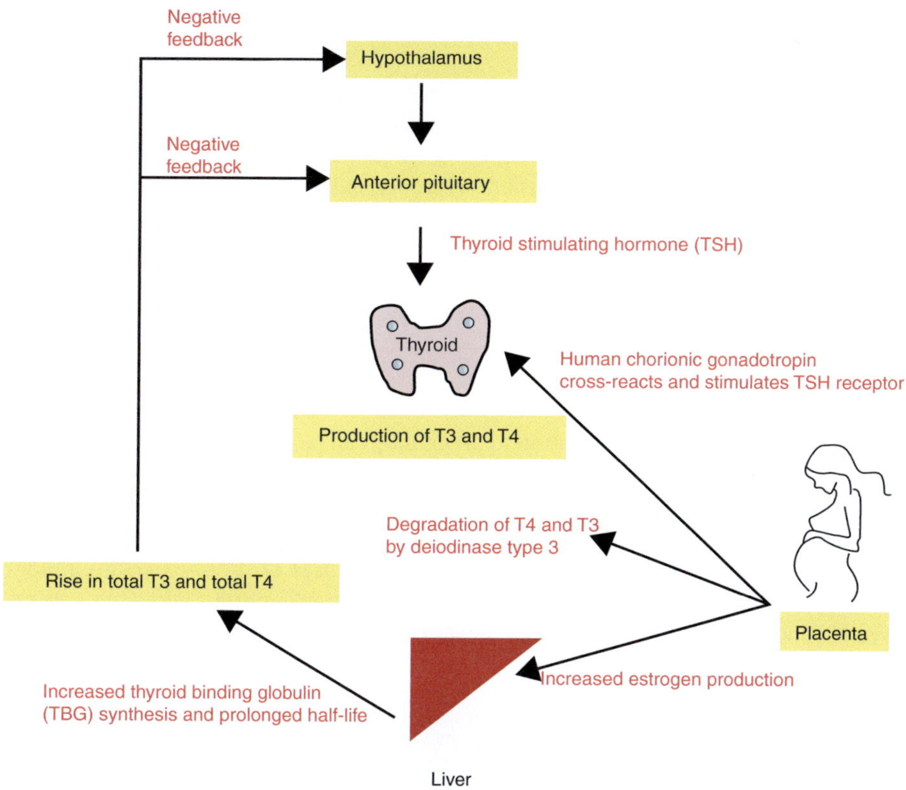

Fig. 6.1 Changes in the thyroid axis in normal pregnancy

6.3 Classification

Hyperthyroidism in pregnancy can be classified biochemically as overt or subclinical. The classification is biochemical and is not based on the presence or absence of symptoms as suggested by the name. Overt hyperthyroidism refers to suppressed TSH below the pregnancy-specific reference range (<0.1mIU/L) with high total or Free T3/T4 for the pregnancy-specific reference range [8]. Subclinical hyperthyroidism refers to suppressed TSH with normal total or free T3/T4 for pregnancy-specific reference range. Total T3/T4 values in pregnancy are 1.5 times the non-pregnancy reference range [8].

6.4 Epidemiology

Although thyroid disease is common during pregnancy, hyperthyroidism is less common and occurs in about 1–2% of pregnancies [9]. Gestational transient hyperthyroidism and Graves' disease (GD) are the most common causes of hyperthyroidism in pregnancy. Gestational transient hyperthyroidism is more common than GD and occurs in the first half of pregnancy in about 1–3% of pregnancies, with higher frequency noted in hyperemesis gravidarum, multiple gestation and trophoblastic disease due to marked elevation of hCG [10].

6.5 Causes

Excess thyroid hormone production in pregnancy can be due to excess TSH receptor stimulation, autonomous thyroid hormone production or extrathyroidal sources of thyroid hormones. The causes of hyperthyroidism are summarised in Table 6.1 [11].

Subacute painful or painless thyroiditis with passive release of thyroid hormones from a damaged thyroid gland are less common causes of thyrotoxicosis in pregnancy, while other conditions such as a TSH-secreting pituitary adenoma, struma ovarii, functional thyroid cancer metastases or germline TSH receptor mutations are very rare.

Table 6.1 Causes of hyperthyroidism in pregnancy

A. Excessive TSH receptor stimulation.
– Graves' disease (TSH receptor autoantibodies).
– Gestational transient thyrotoxicosis (hCG induced).
– Trophoblastic disease and vesicular mole (hCG induced).
– TSH-producing pituitary adenoma.
B. Autonomous thyroid hormone secretion.
– Multinodular toxic goitre.
– Solitary toxic thyroid adenoma.
– Activating TSH receptor mutation.
C. Extrathyroidal sources of thyroid hormones.
– Struma ovarii.
– Functional thyroid cancer metastases.

6.6 Clinical Manifestations

Clinical manifestations of hyperthyroidism may mimic and overlap with those of pregnancy and include palpitations, tremors, heat intolerance and excess sweating. However, the presence of goitre, Graves' orbitopathy, features suggesting congestive cardiac failure, inappropriate weight loss and excessive anxiety should prompt testing for thyrotoxicosis [12]. The specific features of goitre and thyroid eye disease suggest a diagnosis of GD. Conversely, the absence of a prior history of thyroid disease, no stigmata of GD (goitre, thyroid eye disease), a self-limited mild disorder, and symptoms of emesis favour the diagnosis of gestational transient hyperthyroidism [13]. The presence of severe nausea and vomiting may also be encountered in a molar pregnancy, which could be excluded by an ultrasound scan of the abdomen [14].

6.7 Consequences

Mild hyperthyroidism is usually well tolerated during pregnancy and does not have adverse outcomes. Uncontrolled moderate to severe hyperthyroidism can lead to spontaneous abortions, premature delivery, low birth weight, stillbirth, eclampsia and heart failure. Pregnancy can rarely precipitate thyroid storm during labour [15]. 'Foetal programming' is a concept in reproductive physiology that links various exposures during foetal life to the development of disease later in the life of the offspring [16]. Few studies in this regard have shown some association between maternal hyperthyroidism and the development of attention deficit hyperactivity disorder and epilepsy in children [17, 18].

6.8 Approach to Diagnosis of Hyperthyroidism in Pregnancy

A diagnosis of hyperthyroidism in pregnancy is made based on the presence of clinical features as well as laboratory tests. The diagnosis of overt hyperthyroidism during pregnancy is based on the finding of a suppressed (<0.1 mIU/L) or undetectable (<0.01 mIU/L) serum TSH value and a free T4 and/or free T3 (or total T4 and/or total T3) measurement that exceeds the normal range for pregnancy [8]. Once a diagnosis of hyperthyroidism is established, it is essential to differentiate gestational transient hyperthyroidism from GD. Some of the differentiating features of the two conditions are depicted in Table 6.2 [11].

In case of doubt, TSH receptor antibody (TRAb) testing is done. TRAb is positive in 96–97% of pregnant women with hyperthyroidism due to GD [19]. Besides TRAb testing, thyroid ultrasound with Doppler may be performed and this may help in distinguishing GD (high flow) from a subacute or painless thyroiditis (low flow). Its utility in gestational hyperthyroidism is not known. Thyroid radio-nuclide scan, which is usually performed in non-pregnant women to distinguish GD from other

Table 6.2 Comparison of gestational transient hyperthyroidism and Graves' hyperthyroidism[2]

Characteristic	Gestational transient hyperthyroidism	Graves' disease
Time of presentation	First trimester	May be diagnosed anytime, usually in the first trimester
Symptoms and signs	Absent before pregnancy	Might have been present prior to pregnancy
Hyperemesis	More common	No specific relation to hyperemesis
Multiple gestations	More common	No specific relation to multiple gestations
Other manifestations of Graves' disease	Absent	Might be present; e.g. thyroid eye disease, dermopathy
Family history	Usually unrelated	Maybe present
Severity	Usually mild	Any grade of severity may be present
TSH receptor antibodies	Absent	Present
Course	Self-limited	Unpredictable

causes of thyrotoxicosis, is absolutely contraindicated in pregnancy due to radiation risk [19].

6.9 Management

6.9.1 Gestational Transient Hyperthyroidism

Usually, the condition is self-limited and anti-thyroid drugs are not usually required [15]. In case of severe hyperemesis gravidarum, supportive treatment to control nausea and vomiting may be given. Rarely hospitalisation with the administration of intravenous fluids may be required [20]. Thyroid hormones improve gradually as pregnancy progresses. Low-dose beta-blocker (propranolol) may be given in case of severe symptoms. Anti-thyroid drugs are usually not recommended as thyroid function returns to normal by 14–18 weeks of gestation [15].

6.9.2 Graves' Disease in Pregnancy

The aim of treatment is to maintain total T4/free T4 in the high normal reference range for pregnancy. Anti-thyroid drug (ATD) therapy (thionamides) inhibits thyroid hormone synthesis and is the preferred choice in pregnancy. Propylthiouracil (PTU) is preferred in the first trimester as it minimally crosses the placenta and is associated with less frequent and milder foetal defects as compared to methimazole (MMI)/carbimazole (CMZ) [21]. Patients on MMI/CMZ should be switched to PTU if pregnancy is confirmed in the first trimester. After the first trimester, switching to MMI/CMZ may be considered in view of the risk of hepatotoxicity with PTU

[22]. Beta-blockers (Propranolol 10–40 mg thrice a day) may be used in low doses for symptomatic relief.

The initial dose of ATD is based on the severity of hyperthyroidism and symptoms. Initial doses of ATDs during pregnancy are MMI, 5–30 mg/day (usual dose 10–20 mg); CMZ, 10–40 mg/day (usual dose 10–30 mg/day); and PTU, 100–600 mg/day (usual dose 200–400 mg/d). The equivalent potency of MMI to PTU is approximately 1:20 (e.g. 5 mg MMI = 100 mg of PTU). Ten mg of CMZ is rapidly metabolised to approximately 6 mg of MMI. As the half-life of PTU is shorter than that of MMI, PTU dosing should be split into 2–3 daily doses. MMI can generally be given as a single daily dose. In women being treated with antithyroid drugs in pregnancy, free T4 and TSH should be monitored every 4 weeks. The primary goal is to maintain free T4 at a high normal reference range. In a woman diagnosed with GD and on ATD, when found to be pregnant, may opt to withhold medications if clinical and biochemical features are suggestive of remission. Following this, her thyroid function tests may be monitored every 2 weeks in the first trimester and PTU may be initiated if there is evidence of recurrence of disease [8]. An approach to hyperthyroidism in pregnancy is shown in Fig. 6.2.

The details of anti-thyroid drugs are shown in Table 6.3.

MMI, CMZ and PTU cross the placental barrier; thus, ATD therapy for maternal hyperthyroidism also potentially modulates foetal thyroid function. All ATDs tend to be more potent in the foetus than in the mother. Therefore, when the mother is made euthyroid, the foetus is often overtreated leading to hypothyroidism and goitre. In order to avoid a deleterious foetal impact, the aim of treatment is to maintain

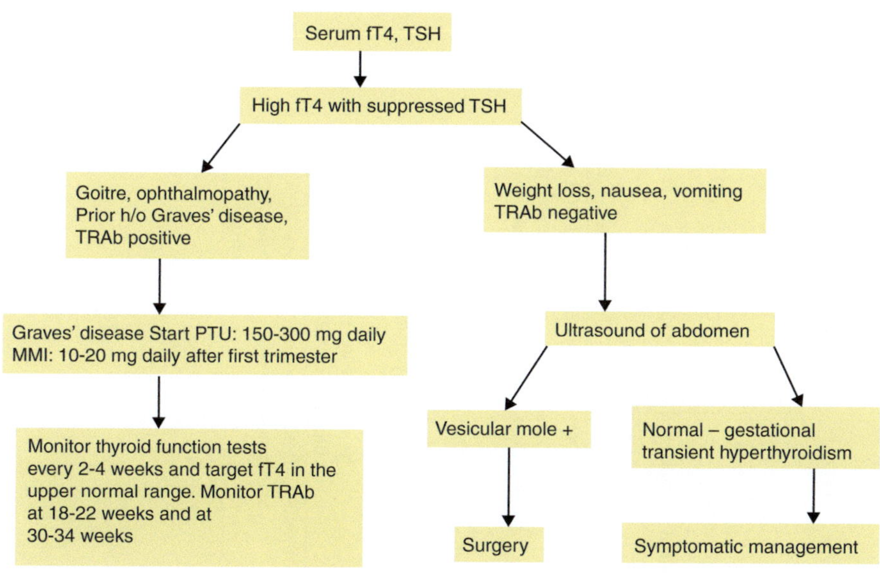

Fig. 6.2 Approach to hyperthyroidism in pregnancy

Table 6.3 Drugs used for hyperthyroidism in pregnancy [5]

Drug	Mechanism of action	Starting dose	Maintenance dose	MMI: Drug potency ratio	General side effects	Embryopathy
PTU	Inhibits thyroxine synthesis, Blocks conversion of T4 to T3	150–300 mg/day, in 3 divided doses	50–150 mg/day, in 2–3 divided doses	1: 20, i.e. 1 mg MMI = 20 mg PTU	Rash Fever Agranulocytosis Hepatotoxicity	Foetal embryopathy less common than with MMI/CMZ
Methimazole	Inhibits thyroxine synthesis	10–20 mg/day	5–10 mg/day	1	Rash Agranulocytosis	Aplasia cutis Methimazole embryopathy
Carbimazole	Inhibits thyroxine synthesis, It is a prodrug, gets converted to MMI	10–30 mg/dl	5–15 mg/day	6: 10	Rash Agranulocytosis	Aplasia cutis Methimazole embryopathy
Propranolol	Reduces adrenergic symptoms	10–40 mg tds, Short-term use only	Short-term use only			Bradycardia, hypoglycemia, preterm birth, small for gestational age

maternal TT4/FT4 values in the high normal range using the smallest possible dose of ATDs [8].

Some of the congenital anomalies that have been variously reported with CMZ include aplasia cutis, choanal atresia, patent vitello-intestinal duct, oesophageal fistula, omphalocele, imperforate anus, microcolon, gall bladder aplasia, ventricular septal defects, hypoplastic nipples, developmental delay and coloboma of the iris or retina [23]. PTU on the other hand is rarely associated with fulminant hepatic failure in the mother. The teratogenic effects associated with PTU use include birth defects of the face and the genitourinary system although these are mild when compared to the teratogenic effects of CMZ [24]. In a recent meta-analysis that consisted of seven studies, it was found that there was an increased trend of congenital anomalies in hyperthyroid women receiving MMI as compared to healthy women in early pregnancy, while the risk was only slightly increased for PTU as compared to healthy women [25]. Thus, it is reasonable to use PTU as the preferred option in women with hyperthyroidism in early gestation.

The combination of levothyroxine (LT4) and an ATD (block-replace therapy) has not been shown to improve the remission rates of GD. This results in a larger dose of ATD required to maintain the FT4 in the target range. As the placenta is more permeable to ATD than LT4, and the foetal thyroid is more sensitive to ATD, this modality of treatment results in foetal hypothyroidism. Thus, the only indication for such combination therapy during pregnancy is in the treatment of isolated foetal hyperthyroidism secondary to maternal TRAb production in a mother who has previously received ablative therapy for GD. The ATD will pass the placenta and treat foetal hyperthyroidism, while the LT4 is required to maintain maternal euthyroidism [8].

Radioactive iodine ablation is absolutely contraindicated in pregnancy due to risk of radiation to foetus. Thyroidectomy in pregnancy is rarely indicated in cases of uncontrolled hyperthyroidism despite maximal doses of ATD or in the presence of severe adverse reactions to ATDs. If required, thyroidectomy should be planned in the second trimester. If there is poor tolerance to ATD, preparation for surgery should include a short course of beta-blockers and 50–100 mg/day of potassium iodide solution. Potassium iodide also helps in reducing bleeding during surgery in case of active thyroid disease. If the maternal TRAb titres are high (> 3 times the upper limit of the reference range), the foetus should be monitored frequently for the development of hyperthyroidism even if the mother is rendered euthyroid post thyroidectomy [8].

The indications for ordering a TRAb test for GD in pregnancy include the following:

(i) The presence of untreated or ATD-treated hyperthyroidism in pregnancy.
(ii) Prior history of radio-iodine ablation or thyroidectomy performed for GD. A value >5 IU/L or 3 times the upper limit of normal in a mother who previously received ablative therapy for GD is an indication for establishing close follow-up of the foetus.
(iii) Previous history of delivering an infant with neonatal hyperthyroidism.
(iv) To distinguish GD from other causes of thyrotoxicosis when detected during pregnancy.

If the TRAb titre done in early pregnancy is found to be low, no further testing is required. If the TRAb in early pregnancy is high, or the woman requires ATD through mid-gestation, a repeat testing is warranted at 18–22 weeks. If the woman continues to be on ATD through the third trimester or elevated levels of TRAb are detected at 18–22 weeks, a repeat testing is required at weeks 30–34 to assess the need for neonatal and postnatal monitoring [8].

6.9.3 Thyroid Storm

Thyroid storm is a rare, but important medical emergency, which can affect <1% of pregnant women with hyperthyroidism. It manifests as acute, severe exacerbation of the symptoms and signs of hyperthyroidism. There is a tenfold higher risk of developing thyroid storm during pregnancy. Precipitating factors include infection, pre-eclampsia, surgery, child birth and induced labour. The diagnosis is based on clinical score of clinical features of raised temperature, cardiac, gastrointestinal, hepatic and neurologic symptoms and signs [26]. Management includes rapid control with PTU, beta-blockers and saturated solution of potassium iodide. Supportive measures include paracetamol and external cooling measures for high temperature, oxygen, intravenous fluids, corticosteroid therapy and management of dyselectrolytemia [27].

6.9.4 Autonomous Nodule

Hyperthyroidism due to an autonomous nodule is rare in pregnancy, and tends to be more insidious and less severe as compared to GD. A major difference from GD is the absence of circulating TRAb in this condition. Thus, there is no stimulation of the foetal thyroid and therefore treatment of the mother to render her euthyroid might result in foetal hypothyroidism. Treatment if warranted is to be restricted to the lowest dose of PTU possible. Surgery for the autonomous nodule may be considered if there develop signs of foetal hypothyroidism [8].

6.10 Foetal Surveillance

Serial ultrasound examinations may be performed for the assessment of gestational age, foetal viability, amniotic fluid volume, foetal anatomy and the detection of malformations. The signs of foetal hyperthyroidism that may be detected on ultrasonography include foetal tachycardia (heart rate > 170 bpm, persisting for over 10 min), intrauterine growth restriction, presence of foetal goitre, accelerated bone maturation, signs of congestive heart failure and foetal hydrops. Serial foetal ultrasound should be carried out once in 4–6 weeks [8].

6.11 Postpartum Period and Lactation

Worsening of disease activity with a need for an increase in ATD dose or relapse of previously remitted disease often occurs after delivery. Women should be informed about this risk, and appropriate monitoring instituted. As far as treatment of GD is concerned, both PTU and MMI can be detected in the breast milk of treated hyperthyroid women. However, only 0.1–0.2% of an orally administered dose of MMI is excreted in breast milk and a woman taking 200 mg thrice daily of PTU secretes 0.149 mg of PTU daily in breast milk; these limits are well below the therapeutic dose [8, 28]. Thus, it may be concluded that the use of PTU or MMI is safe during lactation.

6.12 Pre-conceptional Counselling

Ideally, the choice of therapy in the context of pregnancy should be discussed in all women of the reproductive age group diagnosed to have GD. It is recommended that pregnancy be postponed until a stable euthyroid state (defined as two sets of thyroid function tests in the normal reference range, 1 month apart, with no change in therapy between tests) is achieved. The use of contraception is advisable till thyroid function tests are under control. A woman who wishes to conceive may be offered definitive treatment in the form of ablative therapy with ^{131}I (^{131}Iodine) or thyroidectomy prior to conception [8]. These options may be discussed with the patient in sufficient detail.

Key Messages

- Hyperthyroidism in pregnancy refers to excess thyroid hormone production in pregnancy. Hyperthyroidism should be differentiated from thyrotoxicosis due to excess release.
- Diagnosis of hyperthyroidism can be challenging due to the overlapping symptoms of pregnancy and hyperthyroidism and pregnancy-induced alterations in the thyroid function tests.
- Gestational transient thyrotoxicosis and GD are the two most common causes of hyperthyroidism in pregnancy.
- Gestational transient thyrotoxicosis is usually self-limiting.
- Anti-thyroid drugs are the mainstay of therapy for GD in pregnancy. PTU if preferred in first trimester and CMZ/MMI after first trimester.
- The aim of treatment is to maintain thyroid hormones in the high normal range.
- Free T4 and TSH should be monitored once in 4–6 weeks.

Case Studies

1. A 25-year-old primi gravida presented at 8 weeks of gestation with symptoms of palpitation, excessive tiredness and sweating. There was no prior fever, sore throat, cough or pain in the region of the neck. On clinical examination, she was found to have a heart rate of 94/min, blood pressure of 140/60 mm Hg and a soft goitre. She was noticed to have proptosis and the patient recalled that her eyes had become prominent over the last 4 months. Systemic examination was otherwise unremarkable. Investigations revealed a TSH of 0.008 mIU/L (N: 0.3–4.5 mIU/L), total T4 of 28 mcg/dL (N: 4.5–12.0 mcg/dL) and free T4 was 6.2 ng/dL (N: 0.8–2.0 ng/dL). What is the likely diagnosis and how would you manage this patient?

   Ans:

   This woman presented in the first trimester with clinical and biochemical features of thyrotoxicosis. The presence of a soft goitre with proptosis points to the diagnosis of a GD. The risks associated with uncontrolled hyperthyroidism during pregnancy should be explained to the patient.

   The patient should be initiated on ATD of the thionamide group. PTU is preferred in the first trimester. She may be started on 100–200 mg/day in divided doses with the addition of beta-blockers to control the adrenergic symptoms. Further, she needs to be monitored closely every 2–4 weeks. The dose of PTU is adjusted to target the free T4 in the upper normal range.

   TRAb antibody testing is done, and if found to be high, is re-tested in the second and the third trimester. Foetal surveillance with serial ultrasound scan is undertaken to assess foetal viability, gestational age and the development of foetal thyrotoxicosis.

   After delivery, PTU or MMI may be continued during lactation and dose adjustments may be made according to the results of the thyroid function tests. Prior to her planning a subsequent pregnancy she should be offered definitive treatment for GD.

2. A 31-year-old woman, G2P1L1 presented at 10 weeks of gestation with symptoms of nausea and vomiting. She recalled that she had similar symptoms during her first pregnancy, 8 years back for which she required hospitalisation and administration of IV fluids for recurrent bouts of vomiting. On clinical examination, her heart rate was 90/min and blood pressure was 100/70 mm Hg. There was no evidence of dehydration and there was no goitre. Investigations revealed a haemoglobin of 11 g/dL, creatinine of 0.8 mg/dL and normal serum electrolytes. TSH was 0.013 mIU/L (N: 0.3–4.5 mIU/L), total T4 was 15 mcg/dL (N: 4.5–12.0 mcg/dL) and free T4 was 2.1 ng/dL (N: 0.8–2.0 ng/dL). TRAb was negative. What is the likely diagnosis and the appropriate management?

Ans:

In this case, this woman has gestational transient hyperthyroidism as evidenced by the presence of nausea and vomiting, the absence of goitre and a negative TRAb. She has to be managed symptomatically as this condition is usually self-limiting.

Conflict of interest
Nil.

Funding
Nil.

References

1. Nguyen CT, Sasso EB, Barton L, Mestman JH. Graves' hyperthyroidism in pregnancy: a clinical review. Clin Diabetes Endocrinol. 2018;4:4.
2. Cole LA. Biological functions of hCG and hCG-related molecules. Reprod Biol Endocrinol. 2010 Aug;24(8):102.
3. Soldin OP, Chung SH, Colie C. The use of TSH in determining thyroid disease: how does it impact the practice of medicine in pregnancy? J Thyroid Res. 2013;2013:148157.
4. Fantz CR, Dagogo-Jack S, Ladenson JH, Gronowski AM. Thyroid function during pregnancy. Clin Chem. 1999 Dec;45(12):2250–8.
5. McNeil AR, Stanford PE. Reporting thyroid function tests in pregnancy. Clin Biochem Rev. 2015 Nov;36(4):109–26.
6. Sahay RK, Nagesh VS. Hypothyroidism in pregnancy. Ind J Endocrinol Metab. 2012 May;16(3):364–70.
7. Moleti M, Trimarchi F, Vermiglio F. Thyroid physiology in pregnancy. Endocr Pract. 2014 Jun;20(6):589–96.
8. Alexander EK, Pearce EN, Brent GA, Brown RS, Chen H, Dosiou C, et al. 2017 guidelines of the American thyroid Association for the diagnosis and management of thyroid disease during pregnancy and the postpartum. Thyroid. 2017 Mar;27(3):315–89.
9. Cignini P, Cafà EV, Giorlandino C, Capriglione S, Spata A, Dugo N. Thyroid physiology and common diseases in pregnancy: review of literature. J Prenat Med. 2012;6(4):64–71.
10. Glinoer D. The regulation of thyroid function in pregnancy: pathways of endocrine adaptation from physiology to pathology. Endocr Rev. 1997 Jun;18(3):404–33.
11. Cooper DS, Laurberg P. Hyperthyroidism in pregnancy. Lancet Diabetes Endocrinol. 2013 Nov;1(3):238–49.
12. Grigoriu C, Cezar C, Grigoras M, Horhoianu I, Parau C, Vîrtej P, et al. Management of hyperthyroidism in pregnancy. J Med Life. 2008 Dec;1(4):390–6.
13. Tingi E, Syed AA, Kyriacou A, Mastorakos G, Kyriacou A. Benign thyroid disease in pregnancy: a state of the art review. J Clin Transl Endocrinol. 2016 Dec;6:37–49.
14. Prabhu IK, Rosenbaum A. Hydatidiform mole in a patient with a concern for neoplasia: a case report. Cureus. 2020 Sep 8;12(9):e10319.
15. Moleti M, Di Mauro M, Sturniolo G, Russo M, Vermiglio F. Hyperthyroidism in the pregnant woman: maternal and fetal aspects. J Clin Transl Endocrinol. 2019 Apr;12(16):100190.
16. Andersen SL, Olsen J, Laurberg P. Foetal programming by maternal thyroid disease. Clin Endocrinol. 2015 Dec;83(6):751–8.

17. Nielsen TC, Nassar N, Shand AW, Jones H, Guastella AJ, Dale RC, et al. Association of maternal autoimmune disease with attention-deficit/hyperactivity disorder in children. JAMA Pediatr. 2021 Mar 1;175(3):e205487.
18. Ge GM, Leung MTY, Man KKC, Leung WC, Ip P, Li GHY, et al. Maternal thyroid dysfunction during pregnancy and the risk of adverse outcomes in the offspring: a systematic review and meta-analysis. J Clin Endocrinol Metab. 2020 Dec 1;105(12):dgaa555.
19. Bucci I, Giuliani C, Napolitano G. Thyroid-stimulating hormone receptor antibodies in pregnancy: clinical relevance. Front Endocrinol (Lausanne). 2017 Jun;30(8):137.
20. Nelson-Piercy C. Treatment of nausea and vomiting in pregnancy. When should it be treated and what can be safely taken? Drug Saf. 1998 Aug;19(2):155–64.
21. Ramprasad M, Bhattacharyya SS, Bhattacharyya A. Thyroid disorders in pregnancy. Indian J Endocrinol Metab. 2012 Dec;16(Suppl 2):S167–70.
22. Azizi F, Amouzegar A. Management of hyperthyroidism during pregnancy and lactation. Eur J Endocrinol. 2011 Jun;164(6):871–6.
23. Bowman P, Osborne NJ, Sturley R, Vaidya B. Carbimazole embryopathy: implications for the choice of antithyroid drugs in pregnancy. QJM. 2012 Feb;105(2):189–93.
24. Andersen SL, Olsen J, Wu CS, Laurberg P. Severity of birth defects after propylthiouracil exposure in early pregnancy. Thyroid. 2014 Oct;24(10):1533–40.
25. Li X, Liu G-Y, Ma J-L, Zhou L. Risk of congenital anomalies associated with antithyroid treatment during pregnancy: a meta-analysis. Clinics (Sao Paulo). 2015 Jun;70(6):453–9.
26. Burch HB, Wartofsky L. Life-threatening thyrotoxicosis. Thyroid storm. Endocrinol Metab Clin N Am. 1993 Jun;22(2):263–77.
27. Carroll R, Matfin G. Endocrine and metabolic emergencies: thyroid storm. Ther Adv Endocrinol Metab. 2010 Jun;1(3):139–45.
28. Glatstein MM, Garcia-Bournissen F, Giglio N, Finkelstein Y, Koren G. Pharmacologic treatment of hyperthyroidism during lactation. Can Fam Physician. 2009 Aug;55(8):797–8.

7 Thyroid Nodule and Carcinoma in Pregnancy

T. Parvathi and Arpitha Anantharaju

7.1 Thyroid Nodule

Thyroid nodules are structurally discrete lesions visualised distinctly from the surrounding thyroid parenchyma on various radiological imaging. These nodules may be palpable or non-palpable (detected incidentally during neck imaging for other conditions/"incidentalomas") and can be benign or malignant. As the condition is more common among women of reproductive age group, its detection during pregnancy is challenging for the care provider to rule out the underlying risk of malignancy and its impact on the ongoing pregnancy, also adding anxiety to the expectant mother [1]. A critically balanced approach is necessary for definitive diagnosis and treatment without adversely affecting the obstetric outcome.

7.1.1 Prevalence

A palpable thyroid nodule is the most common clinical finding on routine physical examination. Globally, as per the epidemiological studies, the prevalence of thyroid nodules among women varies from iodine-sufficient (5%) to iodine-deficient (30%) regions, being 4–5 times higher than in men. With the advent of the high resolution Ultrasound (US) and increasing use of various other radiological imaging (carotid duplex studies/CT/MRI/PET) in routine clinical practice, the prevalence of thyroid incidentalomas is 9.4–27%. Table 7.1 highlights the overall prevalence of thyroid nodules in various settings [2–7].

Authors' Contributions: TP and AA have drafted this book chapter.

T. Parvathi (✉) · A. Anantharaju
Department of Obstetrics & Gynaecology, Jawaharlal Institute of Post Graduate Medical Education and Research (JIPMER), Puducherry, India

H. Sagili et al. (eds.), *Thyroid Disease in Pregnancy - A Guide to Clinical Management*, https://doi.org/10.1007/978-981-99-5423-0_7

Table 7.1 Prevalence of thyroid nodules

	Prevalence (%)
In general population	
On clinical examination	3–7
On ultrasound imaging	20–76
Additional nodule on US imaging with one palpable nodule	20–48
In pregnancy	
In mild-moderate iodine-deficient regions	3–21
In severe iodine-deficient regions	30
Risk of underlying thyroid cancer	12–15

7.1.2 Pathogenesis and Risk Factors

- Female sex.
- Elderly age.
- Iodine deficiency.
- Dietary iodine requirements are higher during pregnancy and lactation due to increased thyroid hormone synthesis, urinary excretion of iodine, and foetal iodine requirement. Secondary to these increased demands, 30% of pregnant women in severe iodine deficiency regions can present with thyroid nodules [3].
- Pregnancy and Gestational age.
- Due to various physiological changes noted in early pregnancy, i.e., an increase in the vasculature of the gland and elevated serum human chorionic gonadotrophin (hCG), which mimics thyrotropin hormone, leads to thyroid gland enlargement by 10% in iodine replete versus 20–40% in iodine deficient status along with increasing production of thyroid hormones. In the third trimester, 11–20% of women may experience an increase in the size of the pre-existing nodule along with the development of a new nodule, and 24.4% by 12 weeks postpartum. Studies have reported a doubling of nodule size in 60% of the cases and increased nodular volume [3, 4, 8].
- Parity.
- Multiparity increases the risk of thyroid nodules from 9.4% in nulligravida to 20.7% with previous two pregnancies and 33.9% in women with three or more pregnancies [3, 9, 10].
- History of ionising radiation exposure before 18 years of age.
- History of childhood malignancies involving head and neck irradiation treatment.
- Total body irradiation prior to bone marrow transplantation.
- Family history of benign or malignant thyroid disease.

7.1.3 Clinical Evaluation and Diagnosis

Initial evaluation of thyroid nodules during pregnancy is the same as non-pregnant women:

- Detailed personal and family history.
- Clinical features—Mostly asymptomatic:

- Lump in the neck.
- Compression symptoms such as dysphagia, dysphonia, or dyspnoea.
- Symptoms of hyper/hypothyroidism.
- Physical examination involves focussed inspection and palpation of the thyroid gland and the anterior and lateral cervical nodal compartment for lymphadenopathy. The thyroid gland should be examined for its volume and consistency and record the location of a thyroid nodule, consistency, size, number, and tenderness.
- A thyroid function test (TFT) is to be performed on all pregnant women with a thyroid nodule. In non-pregnant women, a functioning nodule may have subnormal serum TSH levels, which are further evaluated with scintigraphy using technetium pertechnetate or ^{123}Iodine. Rarely functioning or "hot" nodules are malignant and cytologic evaluation can be deferred. However, In pregnancy, scintigraphy is contraindicated, and a physiological decrease in TSH levels, especially in the early trimester, makes it challenging to differentiate between the normal lower levels of pregnancy from functioning nodules [3].
- Ultrasonography (US) of neck.
- It is the most commonly performed initial diagnostic, sensitive, safe, and non-invasive radiological tool for evaluating thyroid nodules. It is indicated in all cases of palpable thyroid nodules, goitre, significant growth in a pre-existing nodule, or symptomatic during pregnancy and with cervical lymphadenopathy.
- Standardised US reporting criteria should be based on the following characteristics of the nodule, i.e., position, size, shape, margins, content, echogenicity, and vascular patterns. It should be focused on risk stratification of malignancy and decision guidance for performing fine needle aspiration cytology (FNAC) for histological diagnosis and further clinical management of the nodule [1]. Standardised US reporting also reduces interobserver variation and effective communication between clinicians, radiologists, and pathologists.
- Based on the US findings, various US classification systems have been proposed to categorise the nodule in either 3 or 5 tiers for the risk of malignancy. They mainly focus on the nodule's pattern-based approach to US imaging.
- In 2017 American College of Radiology (ACR), based on the standard terminology used for US findings and reporting, proposed ACR Thyroid Imaging, Reporting and Data Systems (ACR TI-RADS). Points are given for the US features in the nodules as per the five categories shown in Fig. 7.1. The total points categorise the nodules ACR TI-RADS level ranging from TR1 (benign) to TR5 (Highly suspicious of Malignancy) and thereby guide risk stratification of malignancy and further recommendation for FNAC or US surveillance [11].

Note: The US is not a recommended tool for screening the general population with a low risk of malignancy or with a normal thyroid gland on clinical examination.

- Fine Needle Aspiration Cytology (FNAC).
- A tissue diagnosis is essential to rule out underlying malignancy in the nodule. Decisions for FNAC in the antenatal period should be based on the clinical risk assessment and sonographic patterns for malignancy. It is a safe diagnostic

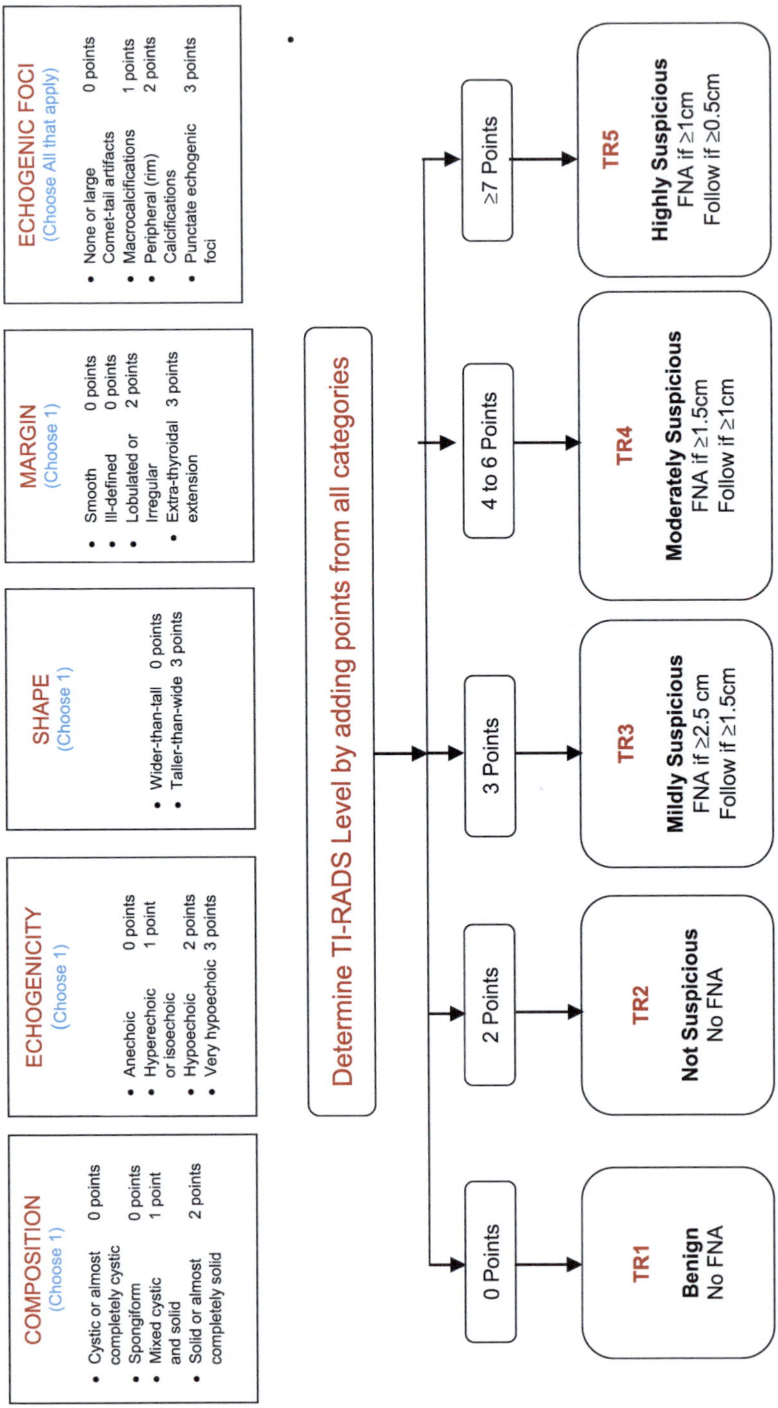

Fig. 7.1 US features and categories as per ACR TI-RADS [11]

Table 7.2 Risk of malignancy (ROM) and clinical management recommendations in a pregnant woman based on FNAC diagnostic category

FNAC diagnostic category	ROM If NIFTP is not malignant (%)	ROM if NIFTP is malignant (%)	Recommended management
I. Nondiagnostic(ND) or Unsatisfactory(UNS)	5–10	5–10	Repeat FNAC, or defer surgery until after delivery
II. Benign	0–3	0–3	Clinical and US surveillance
III. Atypia of undetermined Significance or follicular Lesion of undetermined Significance(AUS/FLUS)	6–18	10–30	Repeat FNAC, or monitor and defer surgery until after delivery
IV. Follicular Neoplasm(FN) or Suspicious for a Follicular Neoplasm(SFN)	10–40	25–40	Monitor and defer until after delivery
V. Suspicious for Malignancy (SUS)	45–60	50–75	Monitor and defer until after delivery
VI. Malignant	94–96	97–99	Surgery in the second trimester or defer until after delivery

modality that can be performed in any trimester of pregnancy. The further decision regarding the timing of the procedure, whether to be carried out during pregnancy or early postnatal period, may be influenced by the underlying malignancy risk and women's preference. As per the ACR-TIRADS criteria, FNAC of the nodules is recommended in the mildly suspicious lesion ≥2.5 cm (TR 3), moderately suspicious lesion if size ≥1.5 cm (TR 4), and in the highly suspicious lesion ≥1 cm (TR 5). Any suspicious-looking cervical lymph nodes on the US or clinical examination should also undergo cytological evaluation. Retrospective case series have reported no cytological alteration of tissue obtained by FNAC during pregnancy [3]. It should always be performed under US guidance to increase accuracy, safety, and reliability and avoid repeat procedures. It can be easily performed using a fine needle of 23- to 27-gauge with accuracy. For satisfactory evaluation, the cytological specimen must have at least six follicles, each containing at least 10–15 cells from two aspirates.

- Thyroid FNA specimen is reported using a standardised category-based reporting system known as The Bethesda System for Reporting Thyroid Cytopathology (TBSRTC). Table 7.2 summarises the TBSRTC's six diagnostic categories with implied risk of malignancy and guides clinicians for further management of nodules in pregnant women [2, 3, 12]. The 2017 revision of TBSRTC also introduced molecular testing for the indeterminate nodule to further reclassify the non-invasive follicular variant of papillary thyroid carcinoma as an adjunct to the cytopathological examination of non-invasive follicular thyroid neoplasm with papillary-like nuclear features (NIFTP) [12]. However, there are no validation studies for its application in pregnant women, and it is currently not recommended for further evaluation of indeterminate nodules during pregnancy [3].

- Serum Calcitonin measurement in all pregnant women is not recommended. It may be measured in women with a family history of medullary carcinoma of the thyroid or MEN 2 or a known RET gene mutation.
- Serum Thyroglobulin levels and Penta gastrin stimulation test are not recommended during pregnancy [3].
- Radionuclide scanning using ^{131}I for evaluation of thyroid nodules is contraindicated during pregnancy. There have been reported cases of inadvertent exposure to ^{131}I during the early trimester where the woman is unaware of her pregnancy. It could be either following evaluation of nodules or for therapeutic purposes with varying doses. ^{131}I readily crosses the placenta and accumulates in the foetal thyroid gland by 12–13 weeks of gestation, causing its destruction and leading to foetal/neonatal hypothyroidism and cretinism. However, these adverse foetal effects have not been reported in exposure prior to 12 weeks of gestation [3, 13]. During the postpartum period, radioactive iodine is concentrated in breast milk. The half-life of ^{131}I is about 8 days which is relatively long, making its use absolutely contraindicated during lactation. Other iodine isotopes (^{123}I) with a relatively shorter half-life of 13 h can be used if deemed necessary for further evaluation of suspected "hot" nodules with suppressed TSH levels. The mother should be advised to pump the breast milk and discard it until the clearance of radioactive iodine from the body, which approximately takes around 3–4 days [3].

7.1.4 Management of Thyroid Nodules

Management during pregnancy depends on the risk of malignancy assessed by the clinical, imaging, and FNAC diagnostic category. Benign nodules during pregnancy are managed similarly to the non-pregnant women with routine clinical and US surveillance. During follow-up, repeat FNAC is indicated in case of rapid growth or suspicious changes in the US for further risk evaluation for malignancy and followed by surgical intervention if required.

- Indeterminate nodules, i.e. AUS/FLUS, SFN, or SUS, in the absence of metastases to neck nodes; surgical intervention can be deferred until delivery. Surgery may be considered during pregnancy in case of clinical suspicion of aggressive behaviour in these nodules.
- Malignant nodules are managed based on the histological type and period of gestation. Surgery should be considered in the second trimester in case papillary thyroid carcinoma diagnosed in early pregnancy showing rapid growth, i.e. 50% in volume and 20% in diameter in two dimensions or presence of metastatic cervical lymph nodes; Differentiated Thyroid Carcinoma (DTC) in advanced stage at diagnosis or medullary or anaplastic carcinoma. If diagnosed in the later half of the pregnancy or case of a stable nodule, surgery can be deferred until delivery.
- Thyroxine suppressive therapy is not recommended during pregnancy for decreasing or arresting the growth of the nodules.

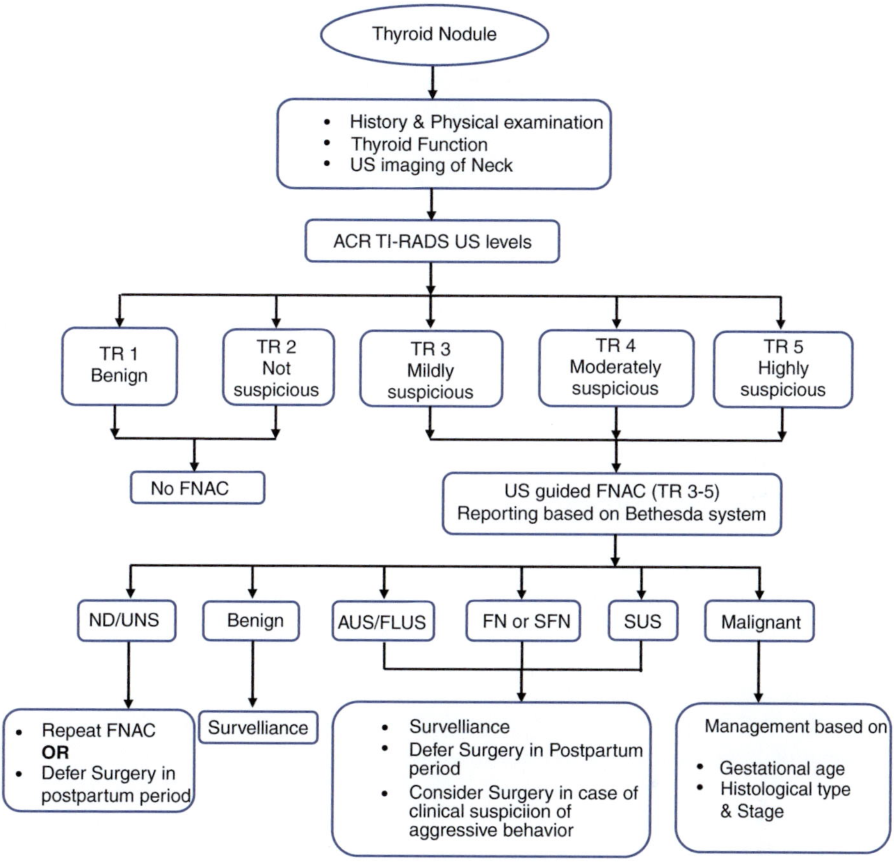

Fig. 7.2 Algorithm summarising the evaluation and management of thyroid nodules in pregnancy. Abbreviations: *ND* Nondiagnostic; *UNS* Unsatisfactory; *AUS* Atypia of Undetermined Significance; *FLUS* Follicular Lesion of Undetermined Significance; *FN* Follicular Neoplasm; *SFN* Suspicious for a Follicular Neoplasm

Figure 7.2 summarises the clinical evaluation, US risk stratification for FNAC, and management of the nodule according to the cytological category.

7.2 Thyroid Cancer

Thyroid cancer is one of the most common endocrine malignancies worldwide. According to the GLOBOCON 2020 database, 586,202 (3%) cases were newly diagnosed, accounting for 43,646 (0.4%) deaths. The global incidence rate is three times higher in women than in men. Age Standardised Rates (ASR) incidence among females varies from 14.3% in the High/Very high Human Development Index (HDI) to 2.6% in Low/Medium HDI countries. Mortality ASR is similar in both High/Very high and Low/Medium HDI countries, i.e. 0.5% [14].

7.2.1 Prevalence

The majority of thyroid cancer cases are present in women of reproductive age. It is the second most commonly detected malignancy during pregnancy following breast cancer, with a prevalence of 14.4 per 100,000 births. The timing of diagnosis during pregnancy is crucial for its management, along with the histological type and stage of the disease. About 3.3 per 100,000 cases are diagnosed in antenatal period, 0.3 per 100,000 at delivery, and 10.8 per 100,000 within 12 months postnatal [3, 5, 8].

7.2.2 Risk Factors

They are similar to risk factors associated with thyroid nodules, as discussed in 7.1.2.

- Age < 20 years or > 70 years.
- Female sex.
- History of thyroid dysfunction.
- Thyroid hormones and TSH are known to cause tumour proliferation through their cell surface reception, oestrogen pathway, increased angiogenesis, and gene expression regulation. Increased risk of malignancy was noted in hypothyroidism (threefold) and hyperthyroidism (4.5 fold) compared to euthyroid individuals. On follow-up for 10 years after diagnosis of hypothyroidism, there was a linear decrease in log risk ratios of thyroid cancer [15].
- Pregnancy.
- The role of sex steroid hormone, i.e. oestrogen, in thyroid carcinogenesis has been hypothesised due to its increased incidence among females than males. Elevated levels of endogenous oestrogen and placental Insulin-like growth factor-I (IGF-I) cause direct growth stimulation of normal and malignant thyroid cells. In cases of newly diagnosed DTC, pregnancy does not increase the risk of cancer progression [16–18].
- History of prior head and neck irradiation treatment <18 years of age.
- Family history of thyroid cancer.
- Hereditary syndromes:
  - Familial medullary thyroid carcinoma (FMTC).
  - Familial papillary thyroid carcinoma.
  - Multiple endocrine neoplasia type 2A and 2B (MEN).
  - Familial adenomatous polyposis (FAP).
  - Cowden's syndrome.
  - Werner's syndrome.
  - Carney complex type 1.
  - McCune-Albright syndrome.
  - DICER 1 syndrome.

7.2.3 Pathology and Molecular Genetics of Oncogenesis

Thyroid carcinoma primarily arises from follicular or parafollicular C cells and is rarely secondary to other malignancies (renal cell carcinoma or local infiltration from carcinoma larynx or oesophagus) [19].

The main histologic types of Primary thyroid cancer are:

1. Differentiated thyroid cancers (DTC) includes papillary, follicular, and Hürthle cell along with their variants.
2. Medullary thyroid carcinoma (MTC).
3. Undifferentiated Anaplastic carcinoma.

Most common histologic type is papillary thyroid carcinoma (PTC) accounting for >90% of all thyroid cancers followed by follicular (4.5%), Hürthle (1.8%), medullary (1.6%), and anaplastic (0.8%) [1, 19, 20].

Mutations in several oncogenes (RET, BRAF, RAS, RET-PTC, PAX8/PPARγ1) and tumour suppressor genes (p53, p16, and PTEN) play a critical role in thyroid oncogenesis. RET proto-oncogene mutation is significantly associated with various types of thyroid cancers. Germline mutations in the RET predispose to MEN 2A, MEN 2B, and FMTCs. Somatic mutations in RET are associated with 30% of MTCs and pheochromocytoma. Rearrangement can cause the fusion of the tyrosine kinase domain of RET with other genes, and the fusion products also function as oncogenes, especially in the carcinogenesis of PTC. At least 15 types of RET/PTC rearrangements have been isolated. RET/PTC3 is associated with a solid variant of PTC and is of aggressive type presenting at a higher stage. RET/PTC, along with other signalling molecules such as Ras, Raf, and MEK, are involved in aberrant activation of the mitogen-activated protein kinase (MAPK) pathway leading to tumorigenesis [7].

RAS gene mutations are found in 20–40% of benign follicular adenomas, increasing their risk of progression to follicular thyroid carcinoma (FTC), papillary and anaplastic carcinoma.

Mutations in BRAF oncogene, most commonly being V600E, are associated with papillary and anaplastic carcinoma. It is not found with a follicular variant of thyroid carcinoma. They usually present with a larger tumour size, an aggressive variant with lymphadenopathy, and local invasion [1, 7].

p53 mutations are rarely found in PTCs but are more common in undifferentiated histology [7].

7.2.4 Staging

Staging is, as per the American Joint Committee on Cancer (AJCC), based on the assessment of the primary tumour(T), regional lymph node(N), and distant metastasis(M).

The primary tumour site(T) is from the thyroid gland's follicular or parafollicular C cells. Rarely, it may arise from the thyroid follicular cells of thyroglossal duct remnants; the thyroid rests in the neck/upper mediastinum (thyrothymic tract) and ovaries (malignant struma ovarii).

The regional cervical lymph nodes(N) are described as per seven-compartment nomenclature. The central neck, i.e. levels VI and VII, is the most common site of nodal metastasis. The lateral neck comprises levels I, II, III, IV, and V. Regional lymph node metastasis can be detected in up to 80% of the cases with PTC. It can also be involved in medullary and anaplastic variants but is less commonly seen in FTC and Hürthle cell cancers.

Distant metastases(M) at the initial presentation are seen in 2–5% of DTC and 1–5% of MTC. Most common site is lung parenchyma (80–85%) followed by bone (5–10%) and brain (1%) [21, 22].

7.2.5 Clinical Features

It mainly presents as an asymptomatic solitary thyroid nodule. During pregnancy, the increase in the nodule size and volume may be noted due to physiological and hormonal changes. The probability of malignancy increases with a rapidly growing nodule, new onset of pain over the nodule, compressive symptoms like dysphagia, dysphonia, or dyspnoea, and physical findings of firmly fixed nodule to the adjacent structures, cervical lymphadenopathy, and vocal cord paralysis [1].

7.2.6 Evaluation and Management

Evaluation is similar to the thyroid nodule as described in Sect. 7.1.3. A thorough workup begins with complete personal and family history, physical examination of the thyroid gland and cervical lymph nodes, and serum TSH measurement, followed by US imaging of the neck for risk stratification of nodules and FNAC of suspicious nodules or lymph nodes [1].

Management of newly diagnosed thyroid carcinoma during pregnancy is challenging. A multidisciplinary team comprising an obstetrician, foetal medicine specialist, endocrinologist, oncologist, radiologist, pathologist, and ENT specialist is essential for comprehensive care of the antenatal mother for optimal maternal, neonatal, and oncological outcomes [5]. Surgery is the definitive treatment. In pregnancy, the timing of diagnosis and histological type of malignancy is crucial for surgical intervention. Post-thyroidectomy maternal risks such as hypothyroidism and hypoparathyroidism should be considered prior to surgery [5]. DTC diagnosed in early pregnancy can be closely followed up with clinical and US surveillance for rapid tumour growth or metastatic lymph nodes. Total thyroidectomy/lobectomy with/without neck lymph node dissection can safely be performed during the second trimester based on tumour size and cervical neck nodal status. Surgery can be deferred for malignancies diagnosed in the third trimester until delivery. No difference was found in recurrence/survival rates following surgery during pregnancy and early postpartum. DTCs have an excellent prognosis with 10-year survival >90–95% [1, 2, 5, 20, 23].

Recurrence/Persistent DTC is of concern in pregnant women. Recurrence or persistence can be diagnosed when stimulated or suppressed serum Tg > 2 ng/ml or increasing Tg autoantibody levels or metastatic cervical lymph nodes in the US and extra thyroid uptake on PET imaging [5]. Routine US and Tg monitoring is not recommended in pregnant women with a history of treated DTC with complete response to therapy. US and Tg surveillance is carried out each trimester in case of high suspicion of persistent structural disease or antenatally elevated Tg levels [23]. In these women, the serum TSH levels should be maintained below 0.1 mU/l. Antenatal mothers need frequent serum TSH level monitoring every 4 weeks to adjust the dosage of Thyroxine [3].

Medullary thyroid carcinoma detected on FNA can be a part of MEN2A or 2B. In pregnant women with RET mutation, excluding pheochromocytoma is recommended before any surgical intervention for MTC. If detected, it should be resected prior to the third trimester, followed by total thyroidectomy with or without neck node dissection for MTC. FDA has approved tyrosine kinase inhibitor (TKI), i.e. sorafenib, lenvatinib, and cabozantinib for metastatic DTC and MTC. All these drugs are found to be teratogenic in animal studies. Each of these drugs has specific advisories. FDA advises counselling for contraception for sorafenib and lenvatinib use and no such specific warning for cabozantinib prescription. Their usage must be guided based on the stage of the disease along with consideration of its risk and benefits [3, 24].

Anaplastic thyroid carcinoma is a rare and aggressive variant with a poor prognosis. It has a median survival of 5 months and 1-year overall survival of 20%. Due to their aggressive nature, they are classified as stage IV by the AJCC TNM system. Management during pregnancy is individualised with the goal of early intervention and coordination among various specialists of the multidisciplinary team [25].

7.2.7 Future Reproductive Outcome

The incidence of thyroid carcinoma is rising, being more common in women of reproductive age. Primary surgery followed by RAI is the standard of care for women with DTC > 1 cm. The use of RAI in adolescents and young adults post-surgically is of concern on future menstrual and reproductive functions.

In the first year of RAI treatment, menstrual irregularities, and amenorrhea were reported in 12% and 8% of the patients, respectively. Effects on ovarian reserve were found to be dose-dependent. RAI dosage of 30–150 mCi significantly decreased the Serum Anti-Mullerian Hormone (AMH) levels by 50% at 3 months following treatment, and only partial recovery was noted at the end of 1 year. At lower doses of RAI, i.e. up to 30 mCi for thyroid remnant ablation, it appears to have an insignificant effect. Women experienced early menopause by 1–1.5 years following ablative therapy. There was no significant increase in adverse pregnancy outcomes like abortion, stillbirths, neonatal mortality, congenital malformation, preterm births, low birth weight, or cancers in the babies. A time interval of >1 year between ^{131}I therapy and pregnancy was associated with a lower risk of abortion than with a < 1-year interval [3, 26, 27]. Therefore, Women undergoing therapeutic RAI are advised to avoid pregnancy for a minimum of 6 months to ensure stable thyroid hormonal function [3].

In cases of MTC with RET mutation carriers, couples should be offered genetic counselling. The options of preimplantation or prenatal diagnostic testing for detecting the mutational status of the embryo or foetus should be discussed. If couples refuse prenatal testing, they should be informed about the availability of genetic testing to detect mutation in their child, especially in the case of MTC before 5 years of age [24].

Clinical Case

A 28-year-old Primigravida, on routine antenatal examination at 12 weeks of gestation is detected to have a palpable thyroid nodule of 2x3 cm, firm in consistency, non-tender, and mobile with a smooth surface. She gives no history of childhood malignancies or head and neck irradiation, and no family history of thyroid cancers.

How do you proceed with further evaluation and management?

A US of thyroid gland and the neck shows a 3.2 × 2.4 × 1.8 cm spongiform lesion, hypoechoic with irregular margins and rim calcifications in the Left lobe. No abnormal cervical lymph nodes are noted. The ACR TI-RADs level was determined to be moderately suspicious (TR4). The US-guided fine needle aspiration cytology of the nodule was reported to be PTC. Serum TSH is 0.5 mU/L. Women was counselled regarding the clinical course of PTC and further surveillance with clinical examination and US were discussed. She was reassured that surgery can be safely postponed until after delivery without increasing the risk of recurrence or survival. If she prefers surgical intervention, it can be safely scheduled in the second trimester without increasing foetal risks. Adjuvant treatment with RAI will be based on the stage of the tumour and if needed will be carried out in postpartum period following further evaluation.

Key Points

- A clinically palpable nodule in pregnancy should be evaluated by ultrasound of the neck and serum TSH levels.
- Based on ultrasound risk stratification of nodule, suspicious lesions must be subjected to FNAC to rule out malignancy.
- DTC diagnosed in pregnancy can be followed up till delivery without increased risk of recurrence or survival.

- In case of rapid increase in size of nodules or appearance of neck nodes or compressive symptoms on surveillance; surgery to be considered in second trimester.
- Surgery is recommended during pregnancy in cases of advanced DTC, MTC, and Anaplastic thyroid carcinoma.
- Genetic counselling with preimplantation or prenatal testing should be offered in couples with RET mutation carriers.

Conflict of interest Nil.

Funding Nil.

References

1. Haugen BR, Alexander EK, Bible KC, Doherty GM, Mandel SJ, Nikiforov YE, Pacini F, Randolph GW, Sawka AM, Schlumberger M, Schuff KG. 2015 American Thyroid Association management guidelines for adult patients with thyroid nodules and differentiated thyroid cancer: the American Thyroid Association guidelines task force on thyroid nodules and differentiated thyroid cancer. Thyroid. 2016 Jan 1;26(1):1–33.
2. Gharib H, Papini E, Garber JR, Duick DS, Harrell RM, Hegedus L, Paschke R, Valcavi R, Vitti P. American association of clinical endocrinologists, American college of endocrinology, and associazione medici endocrinologi medical guidelines for clinical practice for the diagnosis and Management of Thyroid Nodules-2016 update appendix. Endocr Pract. 2016 May 1;22:1–60.
3. Alexander EK, Pearce EN, Brent GA, Brown RS, Chen H, Dosiou C, Grobman WA, Laurberg P, Lazarus JH, Mandel SJ, Peeters RP. 2017 guidelines of the American thyroid association for the diagnosis and management of thyroid disease during pregnancy and the postpartum. Thyroid. 2017 Mar 1;27(3):315–89.
4. Papaleontiou M, Haymart MR. Thyroid nodules and cancer during pregnancy, postpartum and preconception planning: addressing the uncertainties and challenges. Best Pract Res Clin Endocrinol Metab. 2020 Jul 1;34(4):101363.
5. Sullivan SA. Thyroid nodules and thyroid cancer in pregnancy. Clin Obstet Gynecol. 2019 Jun 1;62(2):365–72.
6. Sahin SB, Ogullar S, Ural UM, Ilkkilic K, Metin Y, Ayaz T. Alterations of thyroid volume and nodular size during and after pregnancy in a severe iodine-deficient area. Clin Endocrinol. 2014 Nov;81(5):762–8.
7. Krátký J, Vitkova H, Bartáková J, Telička Z, Antošová M, Limanova Z, Jiskra J. Thyroid nodules: pathophysiological insight on oncogenesis and novel diagnostic techniques. Physiol Res. 2014 Apr;2:63.
8. Wojtczak B, Kaliszewski K, Binko M, Sępek M, Mulek R, Rudnicki J, Bolanowski M, Barczyński M. Thyroid oncology in pregnancy. Annals of Thyroid. Published online. 2020, 5.
9. Angell TE, Alexander EK. Thyroid nodules and thyroid cancer in the pregnant woman. Endocrinol Metab Clin. 2019 Sep 1;48(3):557–67.
10. Zhu J, Zhu X, Tu C, Li YY, Qian KQ, Jiang C, Feng TB, Li C, Liu GJ, Wu L. Parity and thyroid cancer risk: a meta-analysis of epidemiological studies. Cancer Med. 2016 Apr;5(4):739–52.
11. Tessler FN, Middleton WD, Grant EG, Hoang JK, Berland LL, Teefey SA, Cronan JJ, Beland MD, Desser TS, Frates MC, Hammers LW. ACR thyroid imaging, reporting and data sys-

tem (TI-RADS): white paper of the ACR TI-RADS committee. J Am Coll Radiol. 2017 May 1;14(5):587–95.

12. Cibas ES, Ali SZ. The 2017 Bethesda system for reporting thyroid cytopathology. Thyroid. 2017 Nov 1;27(11):1341–6.
13. Iijima S. Effects of fetal involvement of inadvertent radioactive iodine therapy for the treatment of thyroid diseases during an unsuspected pregnancy. Eur J Obstet Gynecol Reprod Biol. 2021 Apr;1(259):53–9.
14. Sung H, Ferlay J, Siegel RL, Laversanne M, Soerjomataram I, Jemal A, Bray F. Global cancer statistics 2020: GLOBOCAN estimates of incidence and mortality worldwide for 36 cancers in 185 countries. CA Cancer J Clin. 2021 May;71(3):209–49.
15. Kitahara CM, de Vathaire F, Boutron-Ruault MC, Journy N. Thyroid dysfunction and cancer incidence: a systematic review and meta-analysis. Endocr Relat Cancer. 2020 Apr 1;27(4):245–59.
16. Rakhlin L, Fish S. Pregnancy as a risk factor for thyroid cancer progression. Curr Opin Endocrinol Diabetes Obes. 2018 Oct 1;25(5):326–9.
17. Troisi R, Bjørge T, Gissler M, Grotmol T, Kitahara CM, Myrtveit Saether SM, Ording AG, Sköld C, Sørensen HT, Trabert B, Glimelius I. The role of pregnancy, perinatal factors and hormones in maternal cancer risk: a review of the evidence. J Intern Med. 2018 May;283(5):430–45.
18. Caini S, Gibelli B, Palli D, Saieva C, Ruscica M, Gandini S. Menstrual and reproductive history and use of exogenous sex hormones and risk of thyroid cancer among women: a meta-analysis of prospective studies. Cancer Causes Control. 2015 Apr;26(4):511–8.
19. Baloch ZW, Asa SL, Barletta JA, Ghossein RA, Juhlin CC, Jung CK, LiVolsi VA, Papotti MG, Sobrinho-Simões M, Tallini G, Mete O. Overview of the 2022 who classification of thyroid neoplasms. Endocr Pathol. 2022 Mar;33(1):27–63.
20. National Comprehensive Cancer Network. NCCN Clinical Practice Guidelines in Oncology (NCCN Guidelines®) for Thyroid Carcinoma V.2.2022. Accessed July 12, 2022.
21. Amin MB, Greene FL, Edge SB, et al. AJCC cancer staging manual. In: Chapter 73, thyroid-differentiated and anaplastic carcinoma. 8th ed. New York: Springer; 2017. p. 873–90.
22. Amin MB, Greene FL, Edge SB, et al. Chapter 74, Thyroid-Medullary. In: AJCC Cancer staging manual. 8th ed. New York: Springer; 2017. p. 891–901.
23. Varghese SS, Varghese A, Ayshford C. Differentiated thyroid cancer and pregnancy. Ind J Surg. 2014 Aug;76(4):293–6.
24. Wells SA Jr, Asa SL, Dralle H, Elisei R, Evans DB, Gagel RF, Lee N, Machens A, Moley JF, Pacini F, Raue F. Revised American Thyroid Association guidelines for the management of medullary thyroid carcinoma: the American Thyroid Association guidelines task force on medullary thyroid carcinoma. Thyroid. 2015 Jun 1;25(6):567–610.
25. Bible KC, Kebebew E, Brierley J, Brito JP, Cabanillas ME, Clark TJ Jr, Di Cristofano A, Foote R, Giordano T, Kasperbauer J, Newbold K. 2021 American Thyroid Association guidelines for management of patients with anaplastic thyroid cancer: American thyroid association anaplastic thyroid cancer guidelines task force. Thyroid. 2021 Mar 1;31(3):337–86.
26. Zhang L, Huang Y, Zheng Y, Cai L, Wen J, Chen G. The effect of I-131 therapy on pregnancy outcomes after thyroidectomy in patients with differentiated thyroid carcinoma: a meta-analysis. Endocrine. 2021 Aug;73(2):301–7.
27. Piek MW, Postma EL, van Leeuwaarde R, de Boer JP, Bos AM, Lok C, Stokkel M, Filipe MD, van der Ploeg IM. The effect of radioactive iodine therapy on ovarian function and fertility in female thyroid cancer patients: a systematic review and meta-analysis. Thyroid. 2021 Apr 1;31(4):658–68.

8 Postpartum Thyroiditis

Swaramya Chandrasekaran and Priyanka Rajandran

8.1 Introduction

Postpartum thyroiditis (PPT) is defined as the de novo onset of thyroid dysfunction, excluding Graves' disease (GD), in a previously euthyroid woman within the first year after delivery. Most of the reported cases of PPT occur after-term pregnancies. As the immunological rebound and postpartum changes after an abortion are similar to term pregnancies some cases of PPT after second trimester miscarriages have also been reported. The prevalence of transient postpartum thyroiditis is approximately between 5 and 10%, while global estimates vary between 1.1 and 16.7% [1, 2]. The wide range in prevalence amongst the general population could be explained by the variations in geographical distribution of women and the study design. PPT is often underdiagnosed owing to the protracted and vague clinical presentation, which may be attributed to the general course of postpartum phase.

Authors' contributions: SC has drafted the chapter. Both authors have reviewed and edited the final manuscript.

S. Chandrasekaran (✉)
Department of Obstetrics & Gynaecology, Sri Venkateshwaraa Medical College Hospital & Research Centre (SVMCHRC), Puducherry, India

P. Rajandran
Department of Obstetrics & Gynaecology, Jawaharlal Institute of Medical Education and Research (JIPMER), Puducherry, India

H. Sagili et al. (eds.), *Thyroid Disease in Pregnancy - A Guide to Clinical Management*, https://doi.org/10.1007/978-981-99-5423-0_8

8.2 Etiopathogenesis and Risk Factors

PPT is considered to have an autoimmune basis central to the development of the condition. Pregnancy is associated with diminished cell-mediated immunity (CMI) and a parallel improvement in immunological disorders during the antenatal period. The rebound recovery of CMI in the postpartum period exacerbates the predilection to immunological disorders as reflected by the onset of PPT. Other mechanisms suggestive of immune mediation include complement activation, natural killer cell activation, T cell changes and a relative fall in cortisol levels due to upregulation of a specific set of cytokines such as Tumour necrosis factor α (TNFα), Interleukin 12 (IL 12) and Interferon ϒ (IFNϒ) and sex steroids postpartum [3]. The autoimmune pathology has been substantiated by multiple indicators like genetic, histological, temporal and clinical which is reinforced by strong clinical correlation with other autoimmune disorders.

8.2.1 Genetic Factors

Thyroid autoimmunity is influenced by a number of genes, those of fundamental significance involving the major histocompatibility complex class I (specific human leukocyte antigen (HLA) haplotypes) are HLA-A1, -BW62, -CW7 and Class II are HLA-DR3, −DR4 and -DR5, in addition to certain other genetic polymorphisms such as CTLA-4 (CT60 cytotoxic T lymphocyte antigen-4). These factors contribute to the prevalence of PPT in women with a family history of hypothyroidism [3] PPT is regarded as a variant form of Hashimoto's thyroiditis due to sharing of HLA-B and HLA-D [4]. Fine needle aspiration cytology (FNAC) of the thyroid gland in PPT shows a dense lymphocytic infiltration, reflecting autoimmune pathogenesis. PPT is differentiated from Hashimoto's thyroiditis by the absence of germinal centres and Hurthle cell changes [5].

8.2.2 Anti-thyroid Antibodies

The best predictor for the development of PPT is TPO-Ab positivity. These antibodies are noted in the first trimester, though only 33–50% of such TPO-Ab-positive women eventually develop PPT. In corroboration, the incidence of PPT in TPO-Ab-negative women is much lower [6]. Furthermore, the titres of TPO-Ab are proportionately associated with the risk of developing PPT; higher the titres, higher the chances of PPT.

8.2.3 Association with Other Autoimmune Disorders

Type 1 diabetes mellitus is associated with increased levels of thyroid autoantibodies, which correlates with the threefold increase in risk of PPT among these women.

Women with pre-existing GD have a higher chance of developing PPT than a flare of GD itself (44 vs 26%) [7]. Other disorders associated with an increase in the risk of development of PPT are Hashimoto's thyroiditis (with residual functional thyroid tissue), systemic lupus erythematosus and chronic viral hepatitis [6].

8.2.4 Other Miscellaneous Factors

PPT is encountered more frequently with smoking, iodine deficiency as well as toxicity, radiation exposure to the neck and intake of certain medications like lithium, amiodarone, Interferon alpha, Interleukin-2 and antiretrovirals [8]. The pathophysiology of PPT is depicted below in Fig. 8.1.

8.3 Clinical Presentation

PPT has varied manifestations, the disease has a characteristic biphasic pattern which marks the classical clinical presentation. The biphasic pattern begins with an initial thyrotoxic phase followed by hypothyroid phase and eventually returns to an euthyroid state [5]. However this pattern is varied and is seen in about 25–40% of women. Isolated thyrotoxicosis and hypothyroidism may be the initial presenting feature in about 20–30% and 40% of women, respectively [6]. The onset of initial phase of the biphasic pattern is triggered by immune-mediated destruction of the thyroid tissue (destructive thyrotoxicosis) leading to a cascade release of stored thyroid hormones and hence, thyrotoxic symptoms. It manifests between 1 and 6 months postpartum, most commonly around the third month, lasting for 1–2 months. The hyperthyroid phase is often only mildly symptomatic, with up to 30% of women being asymptomatic. It may present with a sudden onset, painless goitre and can cause fatigue, irritability, weight loss, palpitations or heat intolerance. In succession, after burn-out of destructive thyrotoxicosis, the patient enters the hypothyroid phase 4–8 months postpartum, peaking at around 6 months and lasting between 4 and 6 months. The hypothyroid symptoms include lethargy, fatigue, cold intolerance, weakness, aches and pains, dry skin, loss of energy and problems with concentration.

Painless goitre can also be seen in PPT during the hypothyroid phase. As thyroid dysfunction has effects on the mood there lies a questionable role of PPT in the development of postpartum depression [5]. The classic form culminates with the recovery of hypothyroid state. Eventually, up to 50% of women go on to develop permanent hypothyroidism [8, 9] (Fig. 8.2).

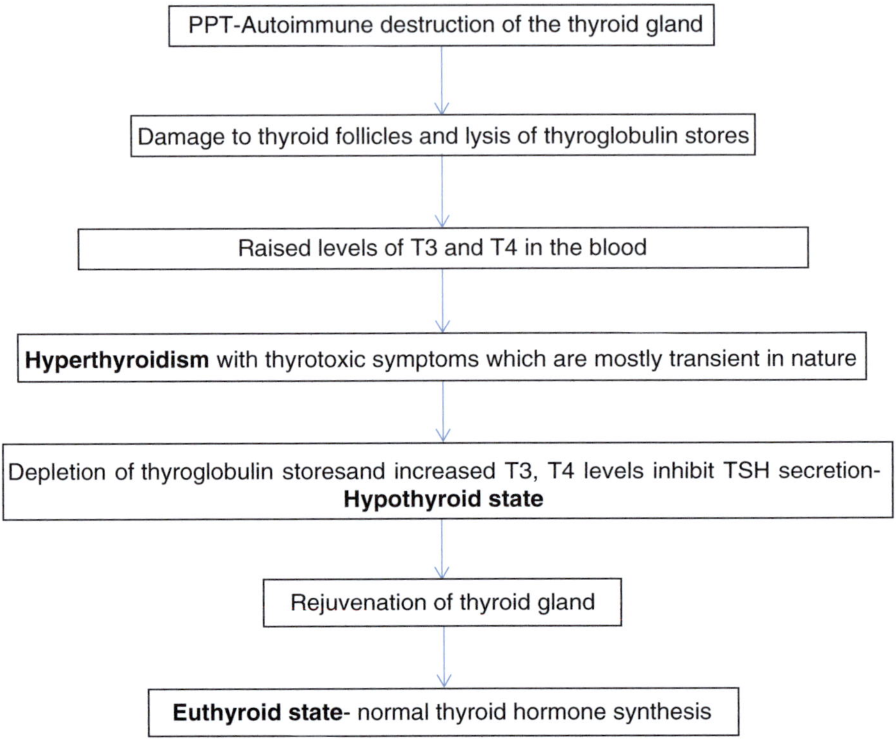

Fig. 8.1 The pathophysiology of PPT

8.4 PPT and Postpartum Depression

Due to rapid withdrawal of hormones in the postpartum period, women are at risk of mood disorders ranging from postpartum blues to postpartum depression (PPD) and psychosis. PPD affects 10–30% of women globally within 1 year postpartum. Studies have shown an association between increased circulating levels of TPO-Ab and the risk of PPD [10]. Thyroid autoimmunity (TPO-Ab positivity) is associated with 1.5 times higher risk of developing PPD in the initial few months after delivery when compared to women who are TPO-Ab negative.

Though the studies linking PPD and PPT have yielded mixed results, PPD could be one of the modalities of presentation in the spectrum of hypothyroid symptoms [11]. Some studies have considered to assess the vulnerability of depression based on the presence of TPO-Ab. TPO-Ab status has been suggested as a possible target in the search for a biomarker to predict the development of mood disorders, such as PPD in susceptible individuals [12]. Therefore it is reasonable to screen women with new-onset PPD, for thyroid dysfunction and TPO-Ab status as hypothyroidism is a reversible cause of depression [13].

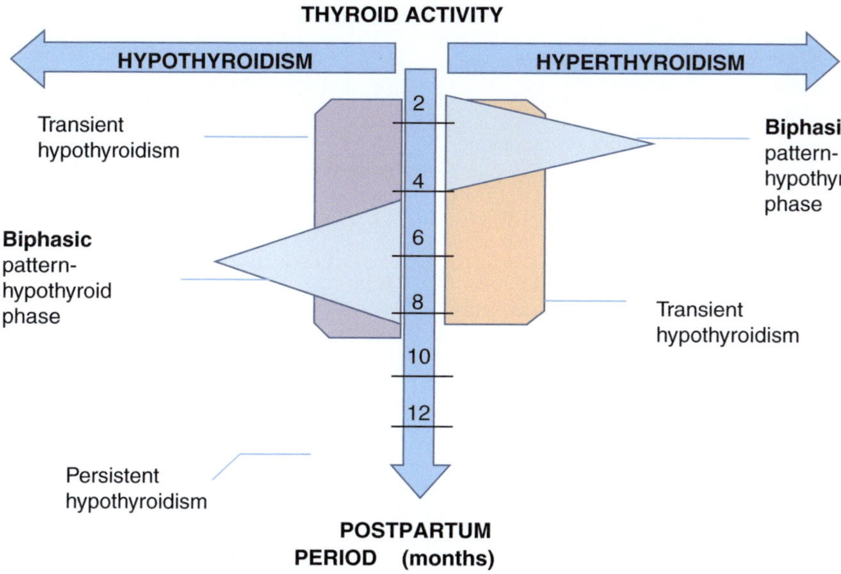

Fig. 8.2 Transient hypothyroidism is the most common presentation (50%), while biphasic presentation and transient hyperthyroidism are noted in 25% each. Around 50% of women with PPT develop permanent hypothyroidism

8.5 Diagnosis

Considering the constellation of symptoms in women with PPT, the diagnosis and decision to investigate is based on clinical discernment. The clinical phase of the disease occurs in continuity. Hyperthyroidism is diagnosed by low levels of circulating thyroid stimulating hormone (TSH) and increased free fractions of triiodothyronine (T3) and thyroxine (T4), while hypothyroidism presents with the contrary. Abnormal levels of thyroid hormones newly diagnosed during postpartum marks the diagnosis of either of the clinical phase of the disease. Though TPO-Ab is not diagnostic, high titres may be found in up to 50% of the women, with 15% showing concomitant thyroglobulin antibody positivity [8]. The timing of onset of disease also gives a clue to the diagnosis and helps in differentiating GD from PPT.

The most common cause of thyrotoxicosis in the postpartum period is PPT and a significant differential diagnosis is GD. The importance of clearly delineating the diagnosis is to define the treatment plan. PPT is treated only if the thyrotoxic symptoms are dominant, more so with beta-blockers alone. On the contrary, GD is treated with anti-thyroid drugs, which is detrimental to PPT, as reflected by the fundamental difference in pathogenesis. Enlisted in Table 8.1 are the differentiating features between PPT and GD [14].

Table 8.1 Differentiating thyrotoxic phase of PPT and Graves' disease

Characteristics	PPT-Thyrotoxic phase	Graves' disease
Likely onset postpartum	1–3 months	Beyond 6 months
Symptoms	Usually mild/ asymptomatic	Overt symptoms. Thyroid bruit and extra-thyroidal features are more common (ophthalmopathy)
Duration of symptoms	Less than 3 months	More than 3 months
FT3: FT4 ratio	Low (increased FT4 due to release of stored hormones)	High
TRAb assay	Negative	Positive
Thyroid ultrasound	Low thyroid volume Variable heterogenous texture, hypoechoic gland/ foci decreased blood flow	High thyroid volume Homogenous echotexture, hypoechoic Increased blood flow (inferno appearance)
Thyroid scintiscan	Low uptake	Elevated uptake

FT3 Tri-iodothyronine; *FT4* Thyroxine; *TRAb* Thyrotropin receptor antibodies

With the availability of more sensitive thyrotropin receptor antibody assays, the need for scintiscan is limited. Should the need arise for definitive diagnosis, isotopes with a short half-life (^{99m}Tc, ^{123}I) are preferred over those with a long half-life (^{131}I), interrupting breast-feeding between 1 and 4 days to minimise infant exposure [5, 14].

When women present with hypothyroidism features, the main differential diagnosis for PPT is Hashimoto's thyroiditis. A definitive diagnosis may be difficult as antibody level measurements may not be useful, owing to an overlap in either condition. Further, the margins of diagnosis are blurred, given that women with PPT could develop permanent autoimmune thyroiditis [5].

8.6 Treatment and Follow-up

Treatment of PPT is limited to symptomatic women and those with specific pregnancy or feeding-related concerns. The thyrotoxic symptoms which occur 2–4 months postpartum resolves spontaneously in most cases. Anti-thyroid drugs such as methimazole and propylthiouracil are ineffective as the symptoms occur due to release of preformed thyroid hormones rather than a rise in production. Symptomatic patients are initiated on lowest possible dose of beta-blockers. Repeat TSH 4–8 weeks after resolution of thyrotoxic symptoms is essential to diagnose hypothyroid phase of the disease. During the hypothyroid phase, treatment is recommended for symptomatic women with TSH between 4 and 10 mIU/L and TSH >10 mIU/L irrespective of the symptoms. In addition, breast-feeding mothers who are symptomatic are also initiated on treatment to maintain a state of euthyroidism [4].

Figure 8.3 represents a schema for the treatment of PPT and the algorithm has been adapted from guidelines of the American Thyroid Association and the American College of Obstetricians and Gynecologists. In women with PPT, annual follow-up with TSH is required as the progression to permanent hypothyroidism is up to 50% with an annual progression rate of 3.6%. Risk factors for progression

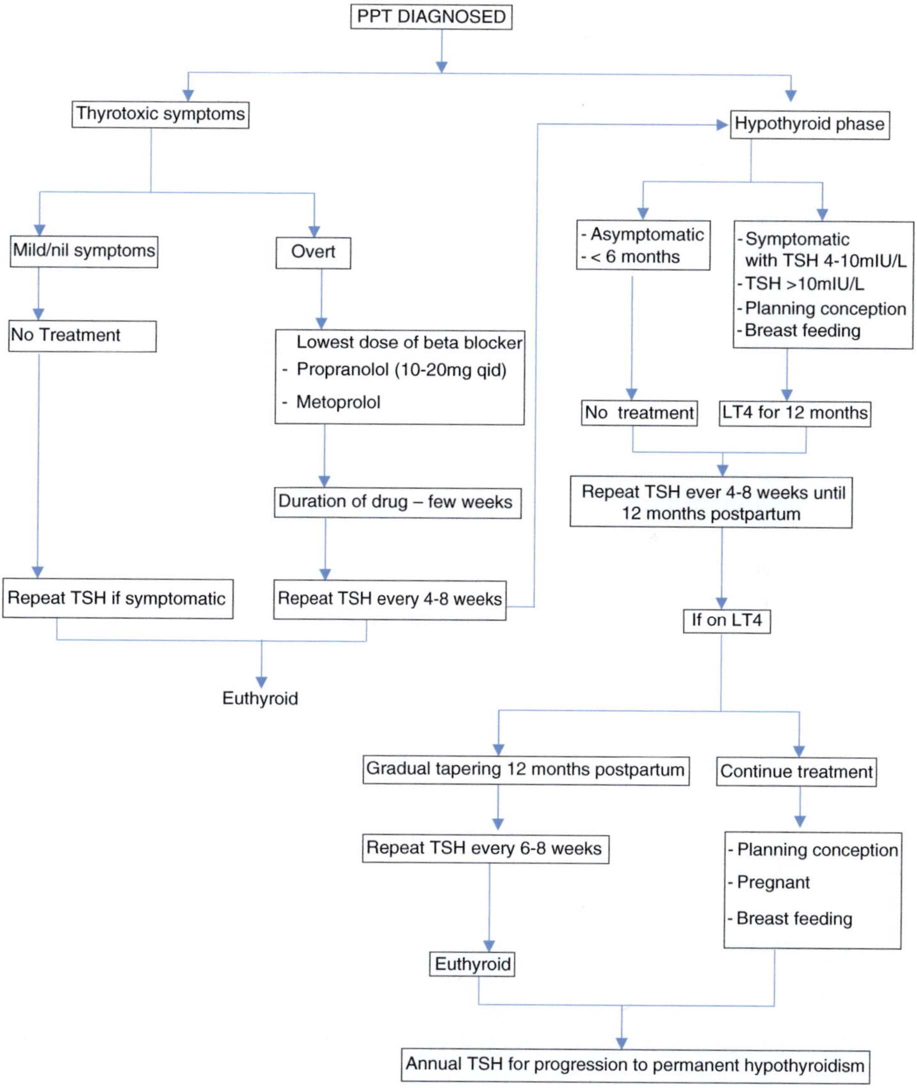

Fig. 8.3 Schema for treatment and follow-up of PPT

include initial high TSH, high titre of TPO-Ab, hypoechogenic gland, family history of hypothyroidism, miscarriage and older women [9, 15].

8.7 Screening for PPT

Universal screening for PPT is not recommended [16]. Women with TPO-Ab positivity in first trimester and those with other risk factors such as autoimmune diseases, genetic predisposition, older age and parity are more likely to develop PPT. The presence of TPO-Ab is the strongest predictor of the disease. Though these factors are not reliable as screening tools, it is suggested that TSH be checked at 3 and 6 months postpartum for women with previous PPT, known autoimmune diseases and chronic viral hepatitis [17, 18].

Euthyroid women with negative TPO-Ab status, testing is not required. Further testing at 6 and 9 months postpartum is required in women who are euthyroid with TPO-Ab positivity [5]. As there occurs risk of permanent hypothyroidism with PPT yearly assessment of TSH is recommended by most of the endocrine societies [9, 12, 16]. High levels of thyroglobulin antibodies, HLA-DR w9 or B 51 among the Japanese population have proven to be risk factors for permanent hypothyroidism [19]. Studies have reported about 70% risk of recurrence in future pregnancies among those who recover from PPT [4].

8.8 Prevention of PPT

Given the propensity for PPT in TPO-Ab positive women, trials have evaluated interventions in lowering the antibody titres with the anticipation of subsequent reduction in the incidence of PPT. Iodine and levothyroxine supplementation in pregnancy have not demonstrated any benefit. Though selenium has shown some benefits, there is an increased risk of development of type 2 diabetes mellitus. The results have not been sufficiently validated to implement routine supplementation. No intervention has been advocated to prevent PPT [20].

8.9 Case Discussion

A 35-year-old woman with a 6-month-old baby and previous 2 miscarriages, presented to her physician with weight gain, generalised fatigue and low mood symptoms. Her pregnancy, delivery and immediate postpartum period were otherwise uneventful. Her mother has type 1 diabetes.

Given the new onset of psychological symptoms in the postpartum phase, with symptoms suggestive of hypothyroidism, TSH, FT4 and TPO-Ab testing is indicated. The woman was subsequently diagnosed with PPT. Additional risk factors include older age, history of miscarriage and family history of autoimmune disease.

Key Messages

1. PPT is diagnosed within the first year postpartum in previously euthyroid women and has an autoimmune basis.
2. TPO-Ab positivity in the first trimester of pregnancy is the strongest predictor of PPT.
3. In classic biphasic disease, the thyrotoxic phase is only mildly symptomatic or asymptomatic. Rarely, when treatment is warranted, beta-blockers are used. Anti-thyroid drugs are avoided. The hypothyroid phase is managed with levothyroxine.
4. Yearly TSH testing is recommended in women who recover from PPT to detect progression to permanent hypothyroidism.
5. No validated preventive measures exist for PPT, though screening of at-risk women is suggested.

Conflict of interest Nil.

Funding Nil.

References

1. Nathan N, Sullivan SD. Thyroid disorders during pregnancy. Endocrinol Metab Clin N Am. 2014 Jun;43(2):573–97.
2. Stagnaro-Green A, Pearce E. Thyroid disorders in pregnancy. Nat Rev Endocrinol. 2012 Nov;8(11):650–8.
3. Tingi E, Syed AA, Kyriacou A, Mastorakos G, Kyriacou A. Benign thyroid disease in pregnancy: a state of the art review. J Clin Transl Endocrinol. 2016 Nov;23(6):37–49.
4. Eaton JL. Thyroid disease and reproduction: a clinical guide to diagnosis and management. Postpartum thyroiditis Springer; 2019:183–188.
5. Samuels MH. Subacute, silent, and postpartum thyroiditis. Med Clin N Am. 2012 Mar;96(2):223–33.
6. Stagnaro-Green A. Approach to the patient with postpartum thyroiditis. J Clin Endocrinol Metabol. 2012 Feb;97(2):334–42.
7. Tagami T, Hagiwara H, Kimura T, Usui T, Shimatsu A, et al. The incidence of gestational hyperthyroidism and postpartum thyroiditis in treated patients with graves' disease. Thyroid. 2007 Aug;17(8):767–72.
8. Argatska AB, Nonchev BI. Postpartum thyroiditis. Folia Med. 2014 Sep 1;56(3):145–51.
9. Thyroid Disease in Pregnancy. ACOG practice bulletin, number 223. Obstet Gynecol. 2020 Jun;135(6):e261–74.
10. Le Donne M, Mento C, Settineri S, Antonelli A, Benvenga S. Postpartum mood disorders and thyroid autoimmunity. Front Endocrinol. 2017 May;4(8):91.
11. Minaldi E, D'Andrea S, Castellini C, Martorella A, Francavilla F, Francavilla S, et al. Thyroid autoimmunity and risk of post-partum depression: a systematic review and meta-analysis of longitudinal studies. J Endocrinol Investig. 2020 Mar;43(3):271–7.

12. Schmidt PMds, Longoni A, Pinheiro RT, et al. Postpartum depression in maternal thyroidal changes. Thyroid Res. 2022;15:6.
13. Bergink V, Pop VJM, Nielsen PR, Agerbo E, Munk-Olsen T, Liu X. Comorbidity of autoimmune thyroid disorders and psychiatric disorders during the postpartum period: a Danish nationwide register-based cohort study. Psychol Med. 2018 Jun;48(8):1291–8.
14. Croce L, Di Dalmazi G, Orsolini F, Virili C, Brigante G, Gianetti E, et al. Graves' disease and the post-partum period: an intriguing relationship. Front Endocrinol. 2019 Dec;10(10):853.
15. Stagnaro-Green A, Abalovich M, Alexander E, Azizi F, Mestman J, Negro R, et al. Guidelines of the American Thyroid Association for the diagnosis and management of thyroid disease during pregnancy and postpartum. Thyroid. 2011 Oct;21(10):1081–125.
16. De Groot L, Abalovich M, Alexander EK, Amino N, Barbour L, et al. Management of thyroid dysfunction during pregnancy and postpartum: an endocrine society clinical practice guideline. J Clin Endocrinol Metabol. 2012 Aug 1;97(8):2543–65.
17. Smith A, Eccles-Smith J, d'Emden M, Lust K. Thyroid disorders in pregnancy and postpartum. Aust Prescr. 2017 Dec;40(6):214.
18. Yalamanchi S, Cooper DS. Thyroid disorders in pregnancy. Curr Opin Obstet Gynecol. 2015 Dec 1;27(6):406–15.
19. Amino N, Arata N. Thyroid dysfunction following pregnancy and implications for breastfeeding. Best Pract Res Clin Endocrinol Metab. 2020 Jul 1;34(4):101438.
20. Alexander EK, Pearce EN, Brent GA, Brown RS, Chen H, Dosiou C, et al. 2017 guidelines of the American Thyroid Association for the diagnosis and Management of Thyroid Disease during Pregnancy and the postpartum. Thyroid. 2017 Mar;27(3):315–89.

MIX
Papier aus verantwortungsvollen Quellen
Paper from responsible sources
FSC® C105338

If you have any concerns about our products,
you can contact us on
ProductSafety@springernature.com

In case Publisher is established outside the EU,
the EU authorized representative is:
Springer Nature Customer Service Center GmbH
Europaplatz 3, 69115 Heidelberg, Germany

Printed by Libri Plureos GmbH
in Hamburg, Germany